Child Protection in Primary Care

Edited by

Janet Polnay

Foreword by

The Minister of State for Health

Dr Ruth Parry
Consultant in Health Policy and Public Health
North Wales Health Authority
IMSCaR
Wheldon Building
University of Wales
BANGOR   LL57 2UW

Radcliffe Medical Press

© 2001 Janet Polnay

Radcliffe Medical Press Ltd
18 Marcham Road, Abingdon, Oxon OX14 1AA

British Library Cataloguing in Publication Data
A catalogue record for this book is available from the British Library.

ISBN 1 85775 224 4

Typeset by Aarontype Ltd, Easton, Bristol
Printed and bound by TJ International Ltd, Padstow, Cornwall

Contents

Foreword

I am pleased to be asked to write a foreword for Dr Janet Polnay's book.

Safeguarding children has been a top priority for this Government since taking office. This commitment has involved new legislation to protect children including the Care Standards Act, Children (Leaving Care) Act and our £885m Quality Protects Programme. But we need to keep this whole issue under the closest continuing review in order to protect vulnerable children and improve professional practice.

The general practitioner's role in safeguarding children is so vital. The GP and other members of the primary healthcare team are often the first to notice when a child is potentially in need of extra help or services to promote health and development, or is at risk of harm. Dr Polnay rightly emphasises that because of their knowledge of children and families, GPs have an important role to play in all stages of child protection processes from sharing information with social services, when enquiries are being made about a child, to involvement in a child protection plan to safeguard a child.

This book is a valuable addition to the literature on child protection. I hope it has a wide readership.

Rt Hon John Hutton
Minister of State for Health
January 2001

Preface

The combination of a general practice background with responsibility for teaching and advising colleagues in child protection has given me valuable insight into the interface between medicine and the agencies involved in protecting children. This book is the result of input from colleagues in the many professions involved in child protection, as well as the desire to pass on knowledge I have gained in a way that I hope strikes a chord with the general practitioner. In the course of doing an MA in child protection, and several case reviews, it became clear to me why there is so often a failure in communication in this important field, and I have been encouraged to pass on what I have learned. The opportunity of working not only with my GP colleagues, but also social workers, the police and other health professionals has been extremely enlightening. As a member of one of the working groups in the revision of *Working Together*, I've been given a unique opportunity to put forward the profession's perspective, as well as learning that of others, with a view to trying to contribute just a little to making the world a safer place for children.

Janet Polnay
January 2001

List of contributors

Janet C Polnay MB BS BSc (Hons) MA
Associate Specialist in Paediatrics
Named Doctor for Child Protection, Nottingham City Hospital
  NHS Trust
Formerly, Principal in General Practice, Nottingham
Medical Advisor, Nottingham Health Authority
Senior Doctor in Child Protection (Primary Care), Nottingham
  Community Health NHS Trust

June Dickens MA RGN RM RHV
Nurse Consultant in Child Protection, Hucknall and Brox-
  towe PCT
Designated Nurse for Child Protection, Nottingham Health
  Authority

Rachel Leheup MB ChB DPM MRCPsych
Independent Child Psychiatrist, Nottingham
Formerly, Consultant Child Psychiatrist, Nottingham Health-
  care NHS Trust

Yin Ng MB BS BSc MD MRCP(UK) FRCPCH DCH DRCOG
Consultant Community Paediatrician, Queen's Medical Centre,
  Nottingham, University Hospital NHS Trust
Designated Doctor for Child Protection, Nottingham Health
  Authority

Michael Page BEM MICPD
Training Consultant
Formerly, Sergeant in Nottinghamshire Police, responsible for
  Child Protection and Interagency Training

David Spicer LLB Barrister
Head of Personal Legal Services, Nottinghamshire County Council

John Thorn BA (Hons) CQSW MSW DMS
Early Years and Partnership Officer, Nottinghamshire Education Department
Formerly, Nottinghamshire Area Child Protection Committee Policy Officer

Acknowledgements

I would like to thank Chris Locke, Nottingham LMC Administrator, without whose idea this book would not have been started, and my husband Leon, without whose encouragement this book would not have been finished. I would also like to acknowledge the other authors for their essential contributions, particularly Yin Ng and June Dickens, who also helped with the planning and content. Thanks are also due to Margaret Harper, BA, MB, BS, DCH, MRCP, MRCPCH, Principal in General Practice, for reading the manuscript and giving valuable feedback.

This book is dedicated to those whose lives
have been marred by abuse

Introduction

This book has been written primarily for general pracitioners, with a view to helping them understand their own and other professionals' roles in the management of child protection. However, all members of the primary healthcare team will find it useful. Other colleagues may also find it helpful to see child protection from the primary care perspective. Whilst acknowledging GPs' difficulties and possible conflicts in this field, the implications of not following the right course of action can be catastrophic and, furthermore, problems may be compounded because these issues are seen relatively infrequently in a normal day's work. This text will help GPs and their primary care colleagues see where they fit in, and how they can contribute to protecting children under their care from abuse and neglect. It has not been the intention to produce a comprehensive reference book for the diagnosis of child abuse, as there are texts available that fulfil that need. The aim has been to explain to GPs the background principles on which child protection management is based, as well as provide a practical 'what to do and why' guide.

1

Child protection in context: Lessons from the past and avoiding common pitfalls

Janet Polnay

Historically, children were viewed as the possessions of their parents, who were at liberty to treat children in any way they wished. In fact, legislation was introduced to protect animals before children were afforded the same 'privilege'. Until recently, corporal punishment at school was deemed by society to be not only acceptable, but necessary, and even today the debate continues as to the appropriateness of smacking children, by parents who seek to enforce discipline. The concept of what is meant by 'child abuse' is thus historically and culturally dependent. In the eighteenth century, children's 'inherent badness' was considered to need disciplining, whilst by the nineteenth century, children's maltreatment had been observed, but was denied. During the twentieth century, legal intervention had at least started to intervene to protect children from abuse. Can we do better in the twenty-first?

The earliest organised professional response to child abuse in Great Britain was the British Society against Cruelty to Children, founded in Liverpool in 1883 (Reder 1993: 13), which led to the NSPCC being established in 1890. However, there has always been debate as to how much the state should interfere with family life. The history of state intervention where there has been concern for a child's welfare has swung between authoritarian state control and respect for family rights (Reder 1993: 16). In 1904, the implementation of the Prevention of Cruelty to Children Act gave local authorities the power to remove children from their parents for the first time.

In 1946, Caffey, a paediatric radiologist in the United States, described bone lesions and subdural haematomas resulting from trauma, and in 1962 Kempe (an American paediatrician) described the 'battered child syndrome' (Kempe *et al.* 1962). Society has been slow to accept that carers could deliberately harm children for whom they are responsible.

The term 'non-accidental injury' (NAI), became the medically accepted label for this syndrome in Britain, and doctors became increasingly involved with social workers and the police in its diagnosis. Medical evidence was necessary for proof, and the traditional medical model methods of history, examination, investigation and diagnosis were appropriate for this initial stage.

Sir Keith Joseph set up the first government departmental guidelines for child abuse management in 1970 and at this time 'at risk' registers were started. Thus, by the 1970s, physical abuse of children had been established as a common occurrence and the beginnings of its management by the medical, social work and police professions had begun.

The death of Maria Colwell in 1974 from physical abuse gave rise to public outcry, and the committee of enquiry that followed stated that 'certain Local Authorities and Agencies in Maria's case cannot escape ... because they must accept responsibility for the errors and omissions of their workers ...' (DHSS 1974: 86). Child protection systems had failed Maria and professionals were blamed for not having done enough. Following this, child protection agencies (all organisations whose work brings them into contact with children and families, including health services, social services, the police, the probation service, education professionals and voluntary organisations) were urged to more effective action and communication to protect children from physical abuse.

Area Review Committees were established following the Maria Colwell enquiry, to review practice, and look at inter-agency co-operation and training issues. Child protection agencies were urged to take more effective action and improve communication to protect children from physical abuse. However, the extent of abuse to children was not, and still may not be, appreciated.

It has been well documented that, historically, children were abused sexually and this was accepted as normal practice. 'The child in antiquity lived his earliest years in an atmosphere of sexual abuse' (De Mause 1994: 43). By the seventeenth century, incest was seen as a crime under church law (Polnay and Hull 1993: 249) and by the time the eighteenth century arrived children were being punished for touching their genitals. The work of Freud, in which patients reported that they had been sexually abused by their parents, was not accepted at the time, probably because of denial in society, and he changed his interpretation to suggest that it was fantasy (Reder 1993: 9, 10). Incest was made a criminal offence in 1908 when the Punish-ment of Incest Act was passed. However, sexual abuse of chil-dren was still thought to be a rare occurrence.

In the 1980s, many papers appeared in the medical press on child sexual abuse. Mrazek et al. (1983) showed that professional recognition of child sexual abuse was at a similar stage to that of physical abuse 20 years ago (Furniss et al. 1984: 865). Sexual abuse of children was simply not talked about, so there was a lack of diagnosis and inadequate treatment. Thus socially and in the medical profession, only in the mid-1980s was the prob-lem of child sexual abuse beginning to be seriously recognised. The actual confirmation of sexual abuse was still seen to be dependent on the medical model, and the role of the doctor seen as the primary one. To compound the problem, society's level of acknowledgement lagged behind that of professionals.

In 1987 a crisis arose in Cleveland resulting in an official en-quiry that was carried out by Lady Butler Schloss (DHSS 1988). Two consultant paediatricians were criticised for diagnosing sexual abuse on the basis of anal dilation, and for splitting up families by admitting many children who were considered to be at risk to hospital. The DHSS circular of 1976 stressed that if a child was suspected of being at risk of a non-accidental injury, that child should be admitted to hospital and the paediatrician would be responsible for its assessment (Parton 1991: 118). These guidelines had enormous implications for the way the children in Cleveland were managed – explaining the multiple hospital admissions.

The Cleveland affair was heavily reported in the press, and for the first time sexual abuse was talked about publicly. Issues causing problems included poor medical and police co-operation, families being torn apart and social services being unable to cope. From the public's point of view, it was necessary to face the occurrence of sexual abuse in our society, and to make matters worse the perpetrators were usually those stalwarts of family life – the breadwinning males.

The report of the Cleveland enquiry had profound implications for the Children Act 1989 (*see* Chapter 2), which was being formulated at the time. Different procedures to be followed when children are physically or sexually abused were developed, and Area Child Protection Committees (ACPCs) were set up. The interests of the child being paramount and the importance of different professions working together were emphasised.

Learning from the past – local reviews

Doctors are well used to, and accept, the format of presenting difficult cases to one another, so lessons can be learned and new management plans formulated. In child protection, the same model is just as valuable but much more difficult to implement, not only because of the number of different professionals involved, but also because of the sensitive nature of the problem. This is where the vital role of the case review (or Part 8 review) (*see* Chapters 2 and 6) comes in to play. The ACPCs, which were set up after the implementation of the Children Act, have the power to call a case review when there has been a child death due to untoward cause or a case of serious injury where abuse or neglect is thought to be a contributory factor, and the case gives cause for concern about professional or inter-agency working. When such case reviews are called, reports are required from all professionals and agencies that have had anything to do with the child and his or her family. The purpose of these reviews is to benefit from experience — to see if the incident could have been prevented, or if current procedures need to be altered to try and prevent further such incidents in the future. Many lessons have been learned from these reviews, and whilst it is appreciated that it is impossible to prevent a parent who is really determined from harming a child, four problem areas regarding professional conduct repeatedly emerge. They are as follows.

Recognition

Failure to recognise abuse may be due to several reasons, ranging from psychological barriers (*see* Chapter 5) to gaps in clinical skills. For example, a professional may not actually recognise that a child has been abused because of an uncommon presentation, e.g. 'deprivation hands and feet' (*see* Chapter 11), observed in cases of neglect, being confused with a cardiac or renal problem. This leads to inappropriate referrals and a subsequent postponement in diagnosis. Delay in recognition may also occur if health visitors or social workers who are carrying out home visits are denied access to a child or excuses such as the child being asleep are accepted. However, a heightened awareness of the occurrence of child abuse can lead to its more frequent recognition.

Communication

As many professionals tend to be involved with families where children are at risk, it is a real problem to enable those involved to have access to all the relevant information. Different professionals coming from different training backgrounds, often speaking in different jargon, is a further complicating issue that must not be underestimated. For example, a situation has arisen where a GP has been absolutely convinced that he made a referral to social services because of concerns about a child, but when a subsequent Part 8 review was carried out, at social services there was no documentation concerning the GP's referral – the communication had been interpreted as a discussion. Unfortunately, the GP omitted to send a follow-up letter to social services confirming his referral. This incident illustrates that GPs need to be very clear in their communications with social workers. Any referral made because of child protection concerns (or, indeed, for any other reason) must be followed up in writing, as is the case when referrals are made to medical colleagues.

One way to improve understanding is to use 'social work language'. If a doctor uses the phrase 'I am referring this child under Section 47 of the Children Act because I am concerned that this child may be at risk of (or has suffered) significant harm', then there is no doubt that a referral is being made because a child is seriously at risk or has already been abused. The words 'significant harm' are words used in the Children Act and Section 47 of the Act carries with it specific duties for social workers in respect of children at risk of harm (see Chapter 9). As social workers are trained to work under statute, once these words are spoken they understand very clearly that they have a statutory duty to carry out an assessment and possibly an investigation. In the same way, a doctor's patients know that if they are worried they are having a heart attack and they ring up and say, 'I have a crushing chest pain going down my left arm', they know they have conveyed the problem immediately to the doctor and can expect an appropriate response. If GPs can learn some of social work's phraseology and use some of the words enshrined in the Children Act, they are more likely to get the response they require from the professional at the other end of the phone. It would improve communication considerably if the professions could learn each other's jargon.

All verbal referrals to social services should be followed up by letter. This is not only good practice, and is no different from that which is expected in a medical setting, but also protects the doctor should any queries be made at a later date.

Procedures

All GPs should be aware of, and have access to, their local child protection procedures (*see* Chapter 3). In some cases, the fact that a child has been at risk has been recognised and good communication has taken place. However, the correct procedures have not been followed and therefore some steps have been missed out. For example, it may be in some cases that a GP has recognised that a child is seriously at risk, or has been abused, and may even have felt that hospital admission was necessary in that particular case, but has *not* made the referral to social services. The GP assumed that the doctor at the hospital would make the referral. However this assumption is fraught with problems. Firstly, the child may not actually arrive at hospital. Thus the child is still at risk and social services have not been informed, but the GP is under the impression that a referral has taken place and all is in hand. Secondly, even though the GP may verbally discuss the problem of the child with the casualty officer, it could be that that very doctor has either gone off-duty or is busy with another patient when the child in question arrives. This means that another doctor who has not had the benefit of the GP's phone call sees the child. These are just two examples where failure to follow correct procedures results in children slipping through the net. The person who is at the first point of clinical contact – in this instance the GP – should usually make the referral to social services. (Consult local procedures.)

Note keeping

Doctors are reminded time and time again by the defence societies how crucial good note keeping is – every set of notes should be kept as if it might need to be viewed in court. Child protection is no exception. Failure to keep adequate notes can mean that a child's life is put at risk. This is particularly important in general practice, when different partners in the practice may see a child. If notes are not clearly and adequately kept, other partners in the practice, or subsequent GPs with whom the child may be registered, will not be aware of risk factors, anxieties and worries. Use of the notes to improve communication in the context of child protection is enlarged upon in Chapter 7.

Over the years, the recognition and handling of child abuse has come a long way. Many lessons have been learnt from tragedies leading to public enquiries, local case reviews and research (DoH 1995). The recent revision of *Working Together to Safeguard Children* (DoH 1999) (*see* Chapter 2) has been strongly influenced by this and recognises that if families can be supported at the stage where they are 'in need' there may be less requirement for child protection action, as potential crises may be averted. There is now much evidence-based information as to how children can be protected from abuse, and it is up to the professions to put into action the knowledge which has been gained.

References

De Mause L (1974) *The History of Childhood*. Bellew Publishing, London.

Department of Health (1995) *Child Protection: Messages from Research*. HMSO, London.

Department of Health (1999) *Working Together to Safeguard Children*. The Stationery Office, London.

Department of Health and Social Security (1974) *Report of the Committee of Enquiry into the Care and Supervision Provided in Relation to Maria Colwell*. HMSO, London.

Department of Health and Social Security (1988) *Report of the Enquiry into Child Abuse in Cleveland*. HMSO, London.

Furniss T, Bingly-Miller L and Bentovim A (1984) Therapeutic approach to sexual abuse. *Archives of Disease in Childhood* **59**: 865–70.

Kempe CH, Silverman FN, Steel BF, Droegmueller W and Silver HK (1962) The battered child syndrome. *JAMA.* **18**: 17–24.

Mrazek PJ, Lynch MA and Bentovim A (1983) Sexual abuse of children in the United Kingdom. *Child Abuse and Neglect.* **7**: 147–54.

Parton N (1991) *Governing the Family*. Macmillan, London.

Polnay L and Hull D (1993) *Community Paediatrics*. Churchill Livingstone, Edinburgh.

Reder P, Duncan S and Gray M (1993) *Beyond Blame*. Routledge, London.

2
The law: *Working Together* and child protection

June Dickens, David Spicer and Janet Polnay

Introduction

The legal responsibility for protecting children from abuse and neglect in this country is held by social services, who have a statutory duty to enquire and take action to safeguard and promote the welfare of children. These important functions cannot be carried out in isolation or in the absence of relevant information and expertise. The legislation therefore provides for social services to have the power to request other professionals and agencies to co-operate and assist with carrying out these functions. The obligation to work collaboratively in this way arises in relation both to individual cases and to planning services.

It is important for GPs working with children and families to understand the relevant legislation, the obligations that this imposes on health services and the implications for professional practice.

The most important legislation underpinning the protection of children is, of course, the Children Act 1989, although there are several other Acts referred to that have relevant provisions for promoting and safeguarding the welfare of children.

This chapter is essentially in two parts. It comprises overviews firstly of the law relating to child protection and secondly of the guidance, *Working Together to Safeguard Children* (DoH 1999) arising from the law.

Philosophy of the Children Act

The Act seeks to balance the need to take effective action to protect children from abuse and neglect with the need to prevent over-intrusive involvement of state agencies in family affairs. It reflects the principle that it is better for most children to be brought up within their families if this is consistent with their welfare. Strong social services powers to take action are balanced by obligations to involve and consult with family members, including children, and to provide a range of services for family support.

Guidance issued by the Secretary of State (DoH 1991a) requires social services to seek to work in partnership with children and families to address their problems. This reflects the principle that if there is agreement on the nature of the problem, agreement on what is to be achieved and agreement on the means to achieve it, the outcome is likely to be more satisfactory. However, the desirability to reach agreement does not override the needs of the child, e.g. if parents do not agree. Section 17 of the Children Act sets out the general responsibilities that local authorities have in respect of safeguarding and promoting the welfare of 'children in need'. (This is described in Chapter 9).

The welfare of the child is paramount when courts are making decisions on a child's upbringing. In making decisions about a child, particularly in relation to care, supervision and contact, the court and others need to be mindful of the 'Welfare Checklist'. This is a list of significant issues to be considered, which includes the fact that the court, in making decisions, should always take into account the wishes and feelings of the child (in the context of her or his age and understanding). Also, courts should only make an order if by doing so it will improve the situation for the child.

Relevant terminology

- The term **accommodated child** refers to a child provided with accommodation (somewhere to live and be cared for) by the local authority or a voluntary agency (e.g. Barnardos) if parents are unable to care, or are prevented from caring, for him or her. The local authority or agency does not acquire parental responsibility (see below) through accommodating the child only. The child may be accommodated in a foster home or children's home, or by some other arrangement.

- A **looked after child** refers to a child accommodated by a local authority, whether or not a care order has been made. The local authority is responsible for developing and implementing a plan to ensure that the child's health, education and social development needs are met.

- **Contact** is the term for access but is wide enough to include, for example, telephone calls or letters.

- **Significant harm** has a particular meaning and establishes a threshold for concern. 'Significant' in this context means noteworthy, which may be through presenting seriousness or presenting implication.

- A **guardian *ad litem*** (GAL) is an independent social worker appointed in childcare proceedings by the court to represent the child's interests in court. Their powers and duties include appointing a solicitor to act for the child and making recommendations to the court about what outcome would be best for the child. The GAL has a legal right to see and make copies of social services records but does not have a right of access to health records (except where they form part of social services records). It is good practice to share information with the GAL, as they are objective and the child's best interests are central to their decision-making. As they are independent practitioners acting on behalf of the court, they provide an important link between the child, the court and other agencies involved in the case.

Parental responsibility

The Act introduced the concept of 'parental responsibility', which is defined as 'all the rights, duties, powers, responsibilities and authority which in law a parent of a child has in relation to their child and his property'. The change in emphasis from parental rights to parental responsibilities was intended to emphasise that children are no longer to be viewed as the property of the parents. It also signifies that parental responsibility diminishes with the increasing age and independence of the child.

Where a child's parents are married to each other at the time of the birth, they each have parental responsibility. Where parents are not married at the time of the birth, parental responsibility rests with the mother. If not married to the mother at the time of the birth, a father may only acquire parental responsibility by court order, by formal registered agreement with the mother, or by marrying the mother. The government's view reflected in a Consultation Paper issued in 1998 (Lord Chancellor's Dept 1998) is that the parental status of unmarried fathers is consistent with Human Rights obligations.

Others may acquire parental responsibility by a residence order (see later in this chapter) being made in their favour by a court. Where an adoption order is made, parental responsibility transfers from birth parents to the adopting couple.

Parental responsibility may be held by more than one person at the same time and can be exercised by one person independently of the others (with a few exceptions). Thus, a medical practitioner may rely on the consent of one person with parental responsibility. The courts decide in cases of disagreement. A local authority acquires parental responsibility (and shares this with the parents who already have parental responsibility) on the making of a care order. However, the local authority may determine the extent to which the parents may exercise their responsibility. Those who have care of a child but no parental responsibility may do what is reasonable in the circumstances to safeguard and promote the welfare of the child.

Private law

The Children Act provides courts with a range of flexible orders that they may use according to the individual needs of the child and family. Section 8 of the Act created four new orders, as follows.

Residence order

This states with whom the child is to live and is the only Section 8 order that may be made when the child is in the care of a local authority. It has the effect of ending any care order and gives parental responsibility to the person with the benefit of the order. If that person is not the parent, then he/she shares parental responsibility with the parents who had parental responsibility prior to the making of the order. Residence may be shared; for example, the child may reside with the mother during term time and with the father in the school holidays.

Contact order

This requires the person with whom the child lives, or is to live, to allow the child to have contact (to visit, stay or correspond) with the persons named in the order.

Prohibited steps order

This prevents the parent(s) of a child, or any other person, taking any step in meeting his/her parental responsibility of a kind set out in the order, without first obtaining the permission of the court. An example may be where a parent is threatening to take a child out of the country without consent.

Specific issue order

This gives directions about the handling of a specific question that has arisen, or may arise, in connection with any aspect of parental responsibility towards a child. The aim of this order is to enable particular disputes between those with parental responsibility to be resolved by the court, e.g. in relation to education or medical treatment of a child. If a child is not subject to a care order but accommodated by the local authority, application may be made for a specific issue order (or a prohibited steps order) to resolve differences between those who have parental responsibility.

Public law

Local authority duty to investigate (Section 47)

The local authority has a statutory duty to make enquiries when it has reasonable cause to suspect that any child in its area is suffering, or is likely to suffer, significant harm, to enable a decision to be made about any necessary action to safeguard and promote the child's welfare. (This is described in detail in Chapter 9.) This means that social services should give serious consideration to a referral from any health professional about a child considered to be at risk. This important statutory duty cannot be carried out without effective and efficient co-operation from others who have relevant opinions and information concerning the child.

Section 47 empowers local authorities to call upon other professionals and agencies to assist them with these enquiries by providing information and advice, and places a duty on those professionals and agencies to assist unless to do so would be unreasonable in all the circumstances of the case. Those agencies include the National Health Services. Social work staff who request assistance under these provisions should be able to explain the reason for the request and the purpose for which any information will be used. However, it is important to recognise that, just as in reaching a diagnosis, it is only the receiver of information who can judge its significance.

This places GPs under an obligation to co-operate with social services and share information, not only about the child but also significant information about parents/carers and other adults who may pose a risk where this is necessary to promote and safeguard the welfare and safety of children (*see* Chapter 7).

When carrying out enquiries, the local authority has a statutory duty to obtain access to the child unless they consider it unnecessary because they have sufficient information. This duty is not subject to permission from those with parental responsibility.

Emergency protection order

Emergency protection orders have replaced the old 'Place of Safety Orders' which were lengthy (28 days) and subject to much criticism. Any person may apply for an emergency protection order, which may be made where the court has reasonable cause to believe that a child is likely to suffer significant harm unless removed from where he/she is, or kept where he/she is (which may include a hospital). The local authority may also apply for an order if, when making enquiries under Section 47, access to the child is required urgently but is being unreasonably denied. It is short, eight days initially, with the possibility of a further extension of seven days only.

Anyone may apply to a magistrate for the order, including a doctor, but usually it will be the local authority, the police or the

NSPCC. It may be granted without notice, but after 72 hours it may be challenged in specified circumstances. The court will give necessary directions, e.g. to enter premises and search for the child (and may include other children believed to be on the premises), to request disclosure of the child's whereabouts, or order medical examinations or contact. Police and other professionals, including doctors, may be asked to assist the local authority to execute the order. The applicant gains temporary, albeit limited, parental responsibility for the child, who may be looked after away from home either in local authority accommodation or in hospital. The child must be returned home as soon as it becomes safe, or, if the situation remains unsafe, renewal or another protective order must be sought before the emergency protection order expires.

Police protection

The police have their own powers under the Children Act to remove a child to suitable accommodation for 72 hours, or alternatively the police may prevent the removal of a child from a safe place, for example, a hospital. The grounds for this would be that the officer must have reasonable cause to believe that a child would be likely to suffer significant harm if action were not taken. This power may also be used to protect runaways, drug users, children whose parents have abandoned them or left them unsupervised and alone, and children found to be living in unhygienic or unsafe conditions.

In situations where abuse or other significant harm is suspected, doctors may need to call on the police to use this power, for example, where young children are found 'home alone', where those with parental responsibility are seeking to remove a child admitted to hospital where this would have serious consequences for the child, or to ensure that a child in need of treatment is sent to hospital from a general practice surgery. The 72-hour duration allows time for further investigation of the child's circumstances and for a court order to be sought where necessary.

The power given is a power to remove or detain, which is quite distinct from a power to enter property. In this respect, it is worth remembering that the Police and Criminal Evidence Act 1984 permits police to enter and search any premises without a search warrant if the proposed intention is to save life or limb. The police may arrest without a warrant any person who has committed any offence where the arrest is necessary to protect a child from that person. They can also obtain a warrant to enter premises and search for children. Social services must be notified when the police have invoked their powers of protection, so that further enquiries can be undertaken and the child placed in appropriate accommodation.

Care and supervision orders

A local authority only has the power to intervene in the care and upbringing of a child against the wishes of a person having parental responsibility where a court has made a care or supervision order in proceedings under Section 31 of the Children Act. Only a local authority or the NSPCC may apply for a care or supervision order. The concept of 'significant harm' is central to any proceedings to protect a child. A court will only consider making a care order or supervision order if it is satisfied that certain 'threshold criteria' of the Act are met. The evidence must establish that the child is suffering or is likely to suffer significant harm, and that the harm is due either to the child not receiving the care that it is reasonable to expect a parent to provide or that the child is beyond the control of the parents. So, not only must the existence or likelihood of significant harm be found, but this must be attributable to the standard of parenting experienced by the child falling below acceptable levels.

Although a care order gives the local authority parental responsibility for the child, it does not remove it from the parents. It becomes a 'shared' responsibility. However, the local authority may have to decide the extent to which the parents exercise their responsibility. As a local authority cannot apply for a residence order, it can only acquire parental responsibility in respect of a child by way of a care order or emergency protection order.

A supervision order may be made if a court decides that there is sufficient concern for a child's welfare to be supervised. The order directs a local authority or probation officer to advise, assist and befriend the child, and allots other specific duties in carrying out the order. This order does not give the local authority or the supervisor parental responsibility; this remains with the parents.

Both care and supervision orders may be made on an interim or temporary basis while the court prepares for a final hearing of the case. Interim orders may include provision for medical or psychiatric or other examinations or assessments to be carried out. If of sufficient age and understanding, the child may refuse to submit to the examination or assessment but this refusal may be overridden by an order of the High Court.

Domestic violence

The links between domestic violence and child abuse are now well known. Research confirms that in England and Wales two women a week are killed by their present or former partners (NHSE 1997). It is important for GPs to be aware that there are legal provisions that may help to secure the safety of women and children.

Part IV of the Family Law Act 1996 sets out provisions for occupation orders, non-molestation orders and Powers of Arrest, and amends the Children Act 1989 to allow the attachment of exclusion orders to interim care orders, and emergency protection orders.

Occupation orders

Briefly, Sections 33—41 outline the terms under which decisions can be made about who should remain in the family home and who can be asked to leave. The issues to be considered will vary depending on whether the occupant is entitled to occupy the property and their relationship to the other party or parties. Occupation orders are not restricted to spouses or cohabitees but may in certain circumstances extend to relatives and joint tenants. When an application is made, the court will have to decide if the risk of harm to the applicant or child in the home justifies an order being made.

Non-molestation orders

Section 42 empowers the court to grant a non-molestation order where it considers it necessary for the protection of a child.

Powers of arrest

Section 47 of The Family Law Act contains a Power of Arrest which may be attached to an occupation or non-molestation order, if it appears to the court that this is necessary to protect the applicant or child.

Exclusion orders

Section 52 and Schedule 6 amended the Children Act 1989 to enable the court, when making an interim care order or emergency protection order, to attach an order excluding a suspected abuser from the home. Such an exclusion order may also have a Power of Arrest attached to it which will enable the police to arrest any person they have reasonable cause to think is in breach of an exclusion order.

Schedule I offences

Schedule 1 of the Children and Young Persons Act 1933 sets out a list of serious offences against a child up to the age of 18 years. This ranges from murder, assault and battery to cruelty (including assault, ill treatment or neglect), sexual abuse, abandonment or abduction. It is important to remember that these offences may be committed by a male or a female. For child protection purposes, those convicted, cautioned, reprimanded or warned for a Schedule 1 offence should be considered to pose a potential risk to children (0–18 years) unless assessed otherwise by social services with the assistance of other agencies – for example, the police and probation service. This is because of the serious nature of the offences. Recent legislation requires those convicted of serious sex offences to register with the police and to notify changes of address.

Human Rights Act 1998

Implementation of the Human Rights Act took place on 2 October 2000 and is applicable to all English courts. The Act implements almost all of the European Convention on Human Rights. The Government has made clear that the Children Act 1989, regulations made under it and guidance relating to child protection have been drafted with regard to human rights principles and that all these instruments are therefore compatible.

Article 2 states that everyone's right to life shall be protected by law and Article 3 states that no-one shall be subjected to torture or inhuman or degrading treatment. Child abuse and neglect may lead to loss of life and is inhuman and degrading. Public authorities are required to carry out their functions in a way that promotes the protection expected to be afforded to children under these articles.

Article 8 provides that everyone has the right to respect for his/her private and family life. It is important to note that there is no *right* to privacy or to family life — the right is to *respect* for these matters. This article requires these issues and the likely impact on them to be properly considered when carrying out public functions.

Any interference with the respect conferred under Article 8 must be in accordance with the law and necessary in the interests of national security, public safety, the prevention of crime and disorder, the protection of health and morals, the protection of the freedoms of others or the economic wellbeing of the country.

The Court of Appeal has considered the impact of Article 8 on the exercise of functions concerned with the protection of the vulnerable and has made it clear that the purpose of the article is to promote protection and not to inhibit it:

> The family life for which Article 8 requires respect is not a proprietary right vested in either parent or child: it is as much an interest of society as of individual family members, and its principle purpose, at least where there are children, must be the safety and welfare of the child. (*Re F* (2000) 3 FCR30)

Far from being a tool to use as an 'opt-out clause' for fear of getting it wrong, human rights legislation may give professionals and agencies even greater leverage to take action to protect children from harm. Having said this, when making assessments of need and risk, professionals should always be mindful of the human rights of everyone involved, including parents, carers and significant family members. The Act really underpins current good practice in working in partnership with parents and carers, and sharing information and concerns with them (unless this would place a child at risk).

All those involved in making decisions about the welfare and safety of children will need to *demonstrate and record* that they have considered relevant issues relating to human rights and that decisions made and actions taken are lawful. For example, GPs may share information with relevant authorities, make referrals to social services or recommend actions to be taken to protect children in circumstances where children are suffering or likely to suffer significant harm, particularly where the harm is preventable or as a result of omissions in care.

All health professionals and organisations have a positive obligation to ensure that respect for human rights is at the core of their day-to-day work and that policies, procedures and practice reflect these principles. It is unlawful to act in a way that contravenes the Act and if this is breached, individuals and organisations may be liable. Although the Act is dynamic, and legal challenges will lead to changes in the interpretation, the basic rights will remain the same.

All GPs should have access to the Home Office-issued guidelines to the Human Rights Act, *Core guidance for public authorities: a new era of rights and responsibilities.*

Working Together to Safeguard Children

The second section of this chapter really arises out of the first and focuses on the guidance *Working Together to Safeguard Children* (DoH 1999), which is produced jointly by the Department of Health, the Home Office and the Department for Education. The 1999 version replaces the previous version of *Working Together under the Children Act 1989* (DoH 1991b). Any copies of the old document still in existence should be discarded.

The Secretary of State for Health and Social Services is empowered to issue guidance to local authorities on how to exercise their social services functions. Local authorities are required to implement the guidance unless there are exceptional circumstances justifying a departure. (Section 7 of the Local Authority Social Services Act 1970). *Working Together to Safeguard Children* has been issued under Section 7.

Working Together to Safeguard Children is particularly informed by the requirements of the Children Act 1989 and also reflects the principles contained within the United Nations Conventions on the Rights of the Child, which was ratified by the UK government in 1991. The document does not have the full force of statute, but should be complied with unless local circumstances indicate exceptional reasons that justify variation.

The following summary, which may serve as a helpful pointer to obtaining information from the main document, is intended to be a brief guide to the content of *Working Together to Safeguard Children*.

Scope and purpose of the document

Working Together sets out how all agencies and professionals should work together to promote children's welfare and protect them from abuse and neglect. It is addressed to all agencies whose work brings them into contact with children and families.

The role of the guidance

It is intended to provide a national framework within which agencies and professionals at local level draw up and agree upon their own more detailed ways of working together.

Section 1: Working together to support children and families

This section emphasises that all children deserve the opportunity to achieve their full potential and describes ways in which this may be achieved. It discusses the shared responsibility of agencies to enable this to happen, and points out the necessity of joint working to safeguard children who are suffering or are at risk of suffering significant harm.

Section 2: Some lessons from research and experience

Lessons from research and experience, and the types of abuse and their impact on children are described. The concept of significant harm is discussed including factors necessary to consider whether this has occurred. The duty of social services under Section 47 is also detailed (*see* above and Chapter 9). Sources of stress for children and families are described. These include the following:

- social exclusion

- domestic violence

- mental illness of a parent or carer

- drug and alcohol misuse.

Section 3: Roles and responsibilities

This section describes in detail the role of the agencies responsible for children. The local authority is charged with responsibility for the establishment and effective functioning of the Area Child Protection Committee – ACPC Forum – which acts as a focal point for local co-operation to safeguard children. The roles and responsibilities in the area of child protection of professionals working within the health service, including GPs and PCG/Ts, are described. *GPs should particularly read this part of the document.*

Section 4: Area child protection committees

The ACPC is an inter-agency forum for reaching agreement about how the different services and professional groups should co-operate to safeguard children in that area and for making sure that arrangements work effectively to bring about good outcomes for children. The document proceeds to describe how this can take effect. It suggests membership of the committee, and this includes representation from the health services.

Section 5: Handling individual cases

This section provides advice on what should happen if somebody has concerns about the welfare of a child or concerns that a child may be suffering or be at risk of suffering abuse or neglect. It sets out clear expectations about the way that agencies and professionals should work together in the interest of children's safety and wellbeing. Although this section is clearly of relevance to all professionals working with children, the chapter points out that other professionals, such as adult mental health workers or substance misuse services, should also consider implications for the children of patients or drug users. Also, when dealing with cases of domestic violence, agencies should consider the implication of the situation for any children in the family.

This section continues by emphasising the following:

- Professionals who may encounter concerns about the wellbeing or safety of the child should know what services are available locally and how to gain access to them.

- Emergency action should never be delayed to protect a child, and concerns about a child's welfare, whether or not further action is taken, should always be recorded in writing. At the close of the discussion, clear and explicit recorded agreement should be reached about who will be taking what action, or that no further action will be taken.

The rest of the section describes individual action step-by-step, depending on different circumstances. Whilst helping to guide health staff as to what action to take, this chapter also describes the role of social services and the police.

Details about case conferences are described and the section emphasises that all those providing information should take care to distinguish between fact, observation, allegation and opinion. An initial child protection case conference (ICPC) is held if agencies judge that a child may continue to suffer or be at risk of suffering significant harm. The ICPC is responsible for agreeing the child protection plan. A core group is set up and has responsibility for the child protection plan.

Summary of timescales

- The initial child protection conference (ICPC) should be 15 working days after the initial strategy discussion, if agencies judge that a child may continue to suffer or be at risk of suffering significant harm.

- The first meeting of the core group formed at the child protection conference should take place within ten working days of the ICPC. The purpose of this meeting is to thrash out the child protection plan, which should set out what work needs to be done, why, when and by whom. The core assessment should be completed within 42 working days of beginning the initial assessment (which is done at initial referral stage).

- The child protection review conference should be held within three months of the ICPC and further reviews should be held at intervals of not more than six months, for as long as the child's name remains on the child protection register.

Section 6: Child protection in specific circumstances

This section focuses on specific circumstances, e.g. children living in residential care, peer abuse, race and racism, bullying, foster care, and action to be taken when allegations of abuse are made against a professional. The particular circumstances of disabled children are also discussed as well as abuse by children and young people. The impact of domestic violence on children is described and possible actions to be taken are mentioned. The particular problems of children involved in prostitution, child pornography and the internet are included.

Section 7: Some key principles

This section discusses working in partnership with children and families, and points out that family members know more about their family than any professional could possibly know and that decisions about children should draw upon this knowledge and understanding. Family members should normally have the right to know what is being said about them and to contribute to important decisions about their lives and those of their children. However, the document also goes on to emphasise that partnership does not always mean agreeing with parents or other family members or always seeking a way forward that is acceptable to them. The aim of child protection processes is to ensure the safety and welfare of the child, and the child's interest should always be paramount.

Sharing information

The document draws on research and experience which illustrates repeatedly that keeping children safe from harm requires professionals and others to share information:

- about a child's health and development
- about exposure to possible harm

- about a parent who may need help, or may not be able to care for a child adequately and safely

- about those who may pose a risk of harm to a child.

Often, it is only when information from a number of sources has been shared, and this is put together, that it becomes clear that the child is at risk of, or is, suffering significant harm.

Paragraph 7.28 (page 80) discusses the fact that 'some professionals and staff face the added dimension of being involved in caring for or supporting more than one family member — the abused child, siblings and alleged abuser. Where there are concerns that a child is or may be at risk of significant harm, however, the needs of that child must come first. In these circumstances the overriding objective must be to safeguard the child.'

The next part of the document discusses in some detail the legal framework of disclosure of confidential information. Issues of confidentiality about children under the age of 16 years are included. *Page 82 — Paragraphs 7.39–7.46 — should be read by GPs. Important issues of professional guidance from the GMC are discussed (and are further explored in Chapter 6 of this book).*

Record keeping

Records should use clear, straightforward language, be concise and be accurate not only in fact but also in differentiating opinion, judgements and hypothesis.

Supervision and support

The document acknowledges that working in the field of child protection entails making difficult and risky professional judgements. All involved should have access to advice and support from peers, managers and named and designated professionals.

Section 8: Case reviews

This section describes the action to be taken when a child dies or is seriously injured and abuse and neglect are known or suspected to be factors. The ACPC should always conduct a review into the involvement with the child and family of the agencies and professionals and consider whether there are any lessons to be learnt from the tragedy about the ways they work together to safeguard children. The chapter describes the purpose of the case reviews, known widely as Part 8 reviews, and emphasises that they are not an enquiry into how a child died or who is culpable, but are to establish whether there are lessons to be learnt, and identify what those lessons are and how they will be acted upon. Neither are case reviews part of any disciplinary process. Management reviews should be undertaken when there is cause for concern, but the criteria for a full case review are not met. All relevant professionals including GPs are expected to contribute reports.

Section 9: Inter-agency training and development

This chapter emphasises the importance not only of making training available to staff in single agency settings but also of the value of inter-agency training.

Conclusion

As stated at the beginning, the aim of this chapter was to give an overview of current legislation and raise awareness of the relevant provisions available to protect children from harm. It is important for GPs to be aware of relevant legislation and guidance, and the implications that these may have for professional practice if they are to work together with other agencies and respond effectively to the needs of vulnerable children and families.

References

Department of Health (1991a) *The Children Act 1989: Guidance and Regulations*. HMSO, London.

Department of Health (1991b) *Working Together under the Children Act*. HMSO, London.

Department of Health (1999) *Working Together to Safeguard Children*. The Stationery Office, London.

Lord Chancellor's Department Consultation Paper (1998) Part II, para. 62.

NHS Executive (1997) Criminal statistics 1992. In: NHS Executive *Domestic Violence*. Department of Health, London.

Additional reading

Allen N (1992) *Making Sense of The Children Act. A Guide for Social and Welfare Services*. Longman Group Limited, London.

Hendrick J (1993) *Child Care Law for Health Professionals*. Radcliffe Medical Press, Oxford.

White W, Carr P and Lowe N (1995) *The Children Act in Practice*. Butterworths, London, Dublin, Edinburgh.

3
Who's who and what's what in child protection?

Janet Polnay

This chapter aims to describe the principal committees and less familiar professional titles concerned with child protection, so that their roles can be appreciated and their help appropriately accessed. As a result, GPs will see that they have an important part to play in child protection management with their own contributions to these sources.

Public inquiries that followed tragedies taken up by the media had a profound effect on the management of child abuse, and Area Review Committees were set up following the death of Maria Colwell in 1973, part of their function being to examine inter-agency co-operation. GPs' importance with regard to detecting children at risk was also recognised in the report resulting from Maria's death (DHSS 1974: 61). In 1988, Area Review Committees were replaced by Area Child Protection Committees (DHSS 1988). The recognition of child protection as the responsibility of many professions has resulted in the creation of several committees that are multi-disciplinary. Important roles, often with titles unfamiliar to the medical profession, have been developed to highlight child protection locally. Duties of such posts include responsibilities for training, advisory facilities and the co-ordination of services. This chapter endeavours to act as a guide through this network and to illustrate its relevance to the GP.

The Area Child Protection Committee (ACPC)

According to government guidance (DoH 1999), there should be an ACPC in every local authority area. Representatives of the main professional bodies responsible for preventing abuse and neglect of children are brought together so that all those involved in the management of child protection problems are in step with one another. The management of a child who has been abused involves many disciplines and it is the ACPC that is responsible for ensuring that agreed arrangements between different groups are enacted effectively.

Unfortunately, local authority, health authority and police area boundaries do not always coincide. This means that in some instances, the ACPC under whose jurisdiction a practice falls may be different from that of the health authority. Also, practices on a border will have patients residing in different local authority areas. Confusion may arise, as local authorities may have slightly differing policies.

Role of the ACPC

The ACPC has many functions, which are described fully in *Working Together to Safeguard Children* (DoH 1999). One of the main tasks of the ACPC is to develop local inter-agency and inter-professional guidelines on procedures in the management of child protection issues. These procedures are the mainstay of co-ordinating child protection work in any particular area and it is the ACPC's duty not only to establish these procedures, but also to maintain and review them at frequent intervals. A further crucial role is that of fostering good working relationships between professions who are involved in working to protect children.

Additionally, the ACPC not only has a commitment to raising standards of professionals' work concerning child protection and to making training recommendations, but also to identifying issues arising from the management of cases and ensuring that any resulting recommendations are implemented.

Accountability

Professionals who sit on the ACPC are accountable to the agencies or professionals that they represent. The participating professional bodies and agencies are therefore responsible together for the actions of their ACPC.

Membership of the ACPC

The exact membership of ACPCs up and down the country varies and depends upon local circumstances and requirements. However, the main services that are concerned with the care of children in any way should be represented. The following have representatives:

- the local authority
- the NSPCC
- the health services (includes managerial and professional)
- the police
- the probation service
- the armed services, where appropriate.

Other members may include:

- someone from the local authority education department
- a variety of other specialists, such as a senior paediatrician, a senior nurse adviser, a child psychiatrist, a lawyer, a local voluntary agency representative, a representative from cultural and religious interests

- a Local Medical Committee (LMC) representative
- an adult mental health professional
- the Crown Prosecution Service

The above list is not comprehensive and exact membership will vary from one ACPC to the next. The medical profession certainly is considered to have an extremely important part to play in ACPCs and this includes GP representation.

Sub-committees of the ACPC

The names of the sub-committees and the exact membership of them will vary from one area to the next. However, as an example, the following list is the framework that Nottingham ACPC follows:

- A training sub-committee – responsible for identification of and overseeing inter-agency training.

- Standards, law and procedures sub-committee – maintains and updates guidance and reviewing protocols.

- Overview sub-committee – considers agency reports on case reviews carried out under Part 8 of *Working Together* (*see* Chapter 2). This sub-committee is also responsible for producing a report on the case reviews.

- Local Child Protection Committee (LCPC) – comprises members of professions who work with children on a local basis. Part of its role ensures effective liaison and collaboration between agencies and professionals within its area. It is particularly valuable in that it is a forum where local professionals can meet and, aside from any formal remit of the committee, can by personal communication begin to understand the roles and problems of colleagues within the child protection field.

Members of LCPCs will often include staff from the NSPCC, social services, the police, the probation service and legal representatives, as well as specialist nurse advisers, GPs, paediatricians, child psychiatrists, and representatives from education and voluntary, religious, cultural and ethnic minority groups. It is a forum where, as well as contributing to the management of child protection, one can learn much from colleagues from different disciplines.

It is sometimes difficult to persuade GPs to sit on ACPC sub-committees (or even ACPCs). This is a great shame, because the more GPs that get involved in child protection and its management, the greater will be the understanding by professional agencies such as social services and the police of the problems that GPs face in their practices, and *vice versa*, and the better co-operation will ultimately be.

Should GPs have problems relating to a specific issue with another professional as regards child protection, they should be aware that they can contact their GP representative on the LCPC (or equivalent), who can then approach the relevant professional to resolve the problem. However, clearly this can only happen if a GP is on the committee in the first place!

The child protection procedures

One of the specific responsibilities of the ACPC is to '... develop and agree local policies and procedures for inter-agency work to protect children, within the national framework provided ...' (in *Working Together to Safeguard Children*). The format of the procedures will vary from place to place, and the book containing the procedures may differ in size and layout. It describes local arrangements for child protection management in the area that the ACPC represents. All GPs should be in possession of an up-to-date version of this document.

The procedures apply to all children under 18 within the area that the ACPC represents. They are binding upon all staff working in the agencies and form a framework within which each person has to make judgements and decisions regarding child abuse.

They are designed to ensure, as far as possible, that all serious harm to children is identified and that the management is carried out in as sensitive a way as possible. The procedures contain information on the procedures and roles of professionals and agencies concerned and also provide an agreed process of co-ordination and collaboration between those agencies (taken from Nottinghamshire ACPC Child Protection Procedures, page 1).

Each set of procedures will have the same principles of managing child protection as are recommended in the document *Working Together to Safeguard Children* (described in Chapter 2). Details, for example, telephone numbers and whom to contact for advice in given situations, will vary from place to place according to local arrangements. The procedures are monitored and revised on a regular basis. They are written and brought together by the representatives of the agencies on the ACPC, and there are specific sections for the medical and nursing professions, as well as for the police, social services and other relevant disciplines. The GP section would usually be written with the main input coming from the LMC representative on the ACPC.

In summary, the procedures are extremely important, and are compiled as a result of statutory direction. They are a result of much discussion, bring together what is established and workable, and should be followed.

Senior professionals who can act as a source of advice to GPs

There is a range of senior doctors and nurses in each ACPC area who can be contacted for advice. Their identity, and indeed the very existence and availability of these doctors, may not be known by local GPs but they can be an invaluable source of help and guidance in child protection matters.

The designated doctor and nurse in child protection

Each health authority identifies a senior doctor and a senior nurse who will take '... a professional lead on all aspects of the health service contribution to safeguarding children' (DoH 1999). The doctor may be a senior community paediatrician, or hospital paediatrician. He/she and the nurse are closely involved with training and case reviews and are able to advise on management. It is clearly useful to know who they are as they are experts in their field and are always prepared to help GPs.

The named doctor and nurse in child protection

Each NHS Trust is responsible for identifying a named doctor and nurse or midwife who '... will take a professional lead within the Trust on child protection matters' (DoH 1999). In hospitals, the doctor is usually a senior paediatrician with a special knowledge of child protection matters. It is therefore useful to know who the named doctor (and named nurse) is for each local hospital Trust as they are also available to guide GPs, although they are mainly responsible for education, training and advice within their own Trust.

Primary Care Groups/Trusts (PCG/Ts)

Primary Care Groups/Trusts are expected to have clear standards for safeguarding children, in accordance with local ACPC protocols, and are also expected to identify a named doctor and nurse or midwife responsible for child protection (DoH 1999).

They may have a child protection representative – whether a GP or health visitor – on their board so that these issues can be addressed, and representation on the ACPC may be shared between the health authority and the primary care groups/ trusts (PCG/Ts). Whatever the local arrangements, the health authority has overall responsibility for ensuring that child protection is adequately provided for by health services.

ACPCs and designated and named professional roles and responsibilities are well established from previous guidance, but the creation of PCG/Ts has led to new guidelines that have far-reaching implications for GPs, and will necessitate a much greater active involvement in child protection than has hitherto been the case. Clinical governance responsibilities also impinge on child protection, and each PCG/T will need to ensure adequate training for all staff in this field.

References

Department of Health and Social Security (1974) *Report of the Committee of Enquiry into the Care and Supervision Provided in Relation to Maria Colwell*. HMSO, London.

Department of Health and Social Security (1988) *Working Together*. HMSO, London.

Department of Health (1999) *Working Together to Safeguard Children*. The Stationery Office, London.

4
A common problem?

Janet Polnay

The true incidence of child abuse is difficult to ascertain for several reasons. A problem must first be defined before it can be quantified, and the perception as to what actually constitutes child abuse varies according to the era under discussion (*see* Chapter 1), from family to family and from one culture to the next. It is not an absolute concept, but: 'it is a socially constructed phenomenon which reflects values and opinions of a particular culture at a particular time' (Gibbons *et al.* 1995).

Corporal punishment in schools – accepted as necessary in Victorian times, but now banned from state schools – is one example of changing attitudes. Whilst physical chastisement within the family is still legal in the UK, undoubtedly the boundaries of what is and what is not acceptable have altered dramatically. Having said that, what some parents clearly feel is normal and necessary verbal or physical admonishment of their children others would consider abusive. Severe physical chastisement that is family-based but not known to others will not be accounted for in figures for physical abuse. In one research study, it was found that 16% of children had received a beating, usually on the leg or bottom, and one in ten children were hit on the head. The severity of punishment was also assessed, and it was found that most were mild but 14% were severe (DoH 1995).

Assessing the incidence of sexual abuse poses its own problems. One study found that three-fifths of women and over a quarter of men surveyed at school or college had experienced minor but unwanted sexual attention when wide-ranging definitions were used. Restricting the definition to physical contact, the prevalence fell markedly. With the most restrictive definition, 4% of females and 2% of males had been sexually abused (Kelly *et al.* 1991). Thus the calculated incidence depends on what is perceived to be abusive. Additionally, the secretive nature of sexual abuse and the fact that it does not 'bruise' must surely mean that much goes on that is not accounted for in official figures.

Neglect is now the most commonly reported category of child abuse (*see* below). It has serious consequences, and offers challenges to the GP. It can be difficult to decide just when a parent's attitude or level of care falls below the threshold that requires intervention. Inevitably, this is influenced by the practitioner's own values, and how much the GP feels these should be imposed on his or her patients. However, it is often difficult to decide what is just about acceptable in terms of growth, development, cleanliness and other aspects of nurturing, especially when the practice is situated in a highly deprived area.

It is almost impossible to estimate the number of children who are emotionally abused, but it has been shown that 3% of children each year are in families who are cold and critical (DoH 1995). Children who are abused in other ways will almost always suffer some emotional abuse.

In addition to the difficulties described above, factors such as variations in reporting and awareness and recognition of child abuse also influence outcomes of attempts to assess the size of the problem. Any figures therefore need to be interpreted with caution.

Rates of abuse

The incidence of abuse is very difficult to measure for the reasons previously discussed. Some idea of the amount of concern over children's safety can be gauged from Section 47 enquiries (*see* Chapter 2). In England per year there are 160 000 such enquiries, including 25 000 which are subsequently unsubstantiated (Gibbons *et al.* 1995). Approximately 25% of referrals lead to initial child protection conferences (ICPCs) and in 1999–2000, 75% of children who were conferenced were placed on the child protection register (CPR). Altogether, about 19% of children who are referred are placed on the CPR. All figures refer to children under the age of 18 years. For the year ending 31 March 2000, there were 30 300 children on the CPR, which represents 27 per 10 000 of the population under 18 years old.

	2000	*1999*	*1998*
ICPCs	38 900	40 800	41 900
Registrations after ICPCs	29 300	30 100	30 000

Table 4.1   Numbers of initial child protection conferences and those that led to registrations 1998–2000 (*Source*: Government Statistical Service 2000).

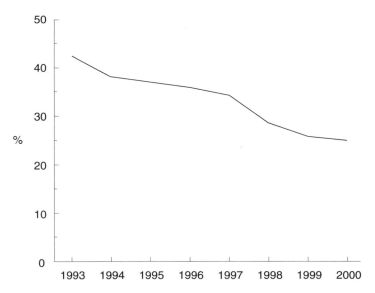

Figure 4.1   Percentage of conferences not leading to registrations during the years ending 31 March 1993–2000 (*Source*: Government Statistical Service 2000).

Length of time on the register

During the year ending 31 March 2000, about 26% (8600 children) had spent less than six months on the register. The number of children on the CPR for more than two years fell sharply between 1994 and 1996 and has continued to fall slowly.

Categories of abuse

The following table illustrates figures from registrations of children on the CPR (showing the mixed categories incorporated in the main categories) in England during the year ending March 2000.

Category	Number	% of total registrations
Neglect	12 900	44
Physical injury	9 500	32
Sexual abuse	5 100	17
Emotional abuse	4 100	17
Categories not recommended by *Working Together*	300	1
No category available	300	1

Table 4.2   Categories of abuse registered during the year ending 31 March 2000 (*Source*: Government Statistical Service 2000).

Some children may be registered in more than one category.

Other estimations put the rate of abuse much higher (National Commission 1996):

Severe physical injury	250 000 annually
Potentially having suffered sexual abuse	100 000 annually
Living in conditions of low warmth and high criticism (neglect, emotional abuse)	350 000 annually

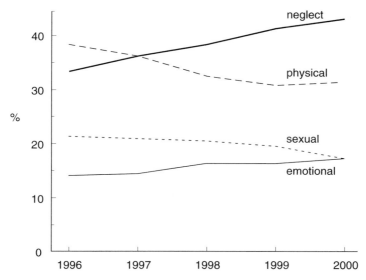

Figure 4.2 Percentage of registrations during the years ending 31 March 1996 to 2000, by category of abuse (including mixed categories) (*Source*: Government Statistical Service 2000).

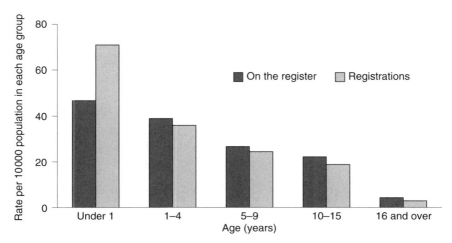

Figure 4.3 Rates of registrations to child protection registers during the year ending 31 March 2000 and rates on the register at that date, by age (*Source*: Government Statistical Service 2000).

Age and gender patterns

Children under one have the highest registration rate (71 per 10 000 children in that age group).

Girls and boys have the same registration rate (25 per 10 000). However, at 31 March 2000, there were slightly more boys on the register; this is because there are more boys than girls in the population aged under 18 (Government Statistical Service 2000).

Characteristics of children and their families dealt with under child protection procedures

Of the 160 000 children about whom enquiries are made annually, the following has been found of them and their families (Gibbons *et al.* 1995):

Characteristic	Percentage of children affected
Headed by lone parent	36%
Both natural parents resident	30%
Dependent on income support	54%
Lacked a wage earner	57%
Domestic violence prominent in family	27%
Mental illness in family	13%
Child previously known to social services	65%
Subject of a previous investigation	45%

Table 4.3 Characteristics of children and their families about whom child protection enquiries are made (*Source*: Gibbons *et al.* 1995).

One in seven parents under suspicion had been abused as a child.

Sources of referral

The major sources of referrals that lead to Section 47 enquiries in Nottinghamshire are:

Source	Percentage
Social workers	16%
Police	15%
School	10%
Parents	10%
Relatives	5%
Health visitors	5%
Self-referrals	8%
Hospital medical staff	3%
Hospital nursing staff	2%

Table 4.4 Sources of referrals that led to Section 47 enquiries (*Source*: Notts ACPC 1998).

GPs account for 2% of total referrals. (Notts ACPC 1998: 31) In contrast, Gibbons *et al.* (1995) found that health visitors, GPs and hospital staff accounted for 17% of referrals (12% in Nottinghamshire).

How are GPs affected by the rates of child abuse?

A GP expects to see a wide range of medical and social problems. Heart disease, chronic lung disease and psychiatric problems as well as upper respiratory infections are amongst the 'bread and butter' of daily surgeries.

How often is the average GP likely to need to deal with a case of child abuse? The answer to this depends on many factors. Considering the attributes of children and families most often referred (*see* Table 4.3), inner city practices are more likely to be involved.

A practice in the inner city areas in Nottingham (City East or City West) is about ten times as likely to have a child on the child protection register compared with a practice in Rushcliffe (which is more affluent) (*see* Table 4.5). There is no reason to believe that this pattern should be different in other areas

	1997	1998	Percent change	Number per 1000 children under the age of 18 at 31 March 1998
Ashfield	113	106	−6%	4.1
Bassetlaw	38	67	76%	2.8
Broxtowe	40	51	28%	2.3
City East	138	178	29%	5.7
City West	256	268	5%	6.5
Gedling	19	24	26%	1.0
Mansfield	71	110	55%	4.5
Newark	42	43	2%	1.9
Rushcliffe	18	16	−11%	0.7
Nottinghamshire	**735**	**863**	**17%**	**3.6**

Table 4.5 Numbers of children on the child protection register as at 31 March 1998 (*Source*: Notts ACPC 1998).

of the country. If a practice has 1000 patients under the age of 18 years, an inner city practice would have between 6.4 and 7.4 children on the register at any one time, while a practice in a more affluent area would have 0.7 children per 1000 on the register.

However, recognition depends also on the level of awareness of the GP and the primary healthcare team. Child abuse takes place in all strata of society and much is undoubtedly missed, especially in the more affluent areas.

In those practices where child protection problems are infrequent, not only may the level of awareness be lower (possibly leading to children at risk being missed), but also, when a case of child abuse does occur, practices may be less familiar with the correct course of action. The GP manages common problems routinely, and when complications arise, local paths of referral or sources of advice are familiar and easily accessed. However, when a rarely encountered problem arises, important telephone numbers may not be at hand, local procedures may not be immediately available for reference and, particularly in the highly charged circumstances that child protection engenders, the whole process is more difficult.

What is certain is that a GP will have to deal with a child protection situation at some time in his or her career. It is the responsibility of the GP to ensure that the primary healthcare team is trained and aware of the issues involved. It is very important that practices know whom they can contact locally for advice on a 24-hour basis, have social services phone numbers for child protection referrals easily accessible and have up-to-date child protection procedures easily to hand. The consequences of not knowing what to do or failure to recognise when children are at risk of significant harm can be far-reaching. At the extreme, a child death could occur, with all the guilt that then ensues. Failure to follow correct procedures may come to light in a case review and the practice is then left feeling it could have done better. Although child protection protocols within the practice may be improved as a result, it is better to be well-prepared initially.

Familiarity with the appropriate management of child abuse is clearly in the GP's and the child's best interests, even though child protection problems are much less common than other aspects of general practice.

References

Department of Health (1995) *Child Protection: Messages from Research*. HMSO, London.

Gibbons J, Conroy S and Bell C (1995) *Operating the Child Protection System: A Study of Child Protection Practices in English Local Authorities*. HMSO, London.

Government Statistical Service (2000) *Children and Young People on Child Protection Registers Year Ending 31 March 2000*. Government Statistical Service, London.

Kelly L, Regan L and Burton S (1991) *An Exploratory Study of the Prevalence of Sexual Abuse in a Sample of 16–21 Year Olds*.

Child and Woman Abuse Studies Unit, University of North London, London.

National Commission of Inquiry into the Prevention of Child Abuse (1996) *Childhood Matters Volume 1.* HMSO, London.

Nottinghamshire Area Child Protection Committee (1998) *Annual Report 1997–1998.* Notts ACPC, Nottingham.

5
Why child protection management is different from other medical problems

Janet Polnay

Dealing with a case of child abuse engenders many emotions. Practical and psychological barriers need to be overcome for its appropriate management, because many basic premises of medical practice are different when applied to a child protection issue. This can lead to confusion, and may result in mistakes occurring. The purpose of this chapter is to highlight some of these issues, as increased understanding of any problem helps the avoidance of potential pitfalls.

The relationship between children and their parents

It is natural and automatic for doctors to believe that parents have the best interests of their child at heart, so the systematic harming or even murder of a child is beyond a doctor's (and most people's) comprehension. The need to 'think the unthinkable' is brought into play and, not surprisingly, it is very difficult to come to terms with the fact that parents can inflict this kind of harm on children. One of the biggest barriers to the recognition of child abuse is the acceptance that it can happen at all, and, moreover, the realisation that a patient who has possibly been known to the practice for many years could be a perpetrator.

Putting the patient first – but which patient?

General practitioners are used to obtaining the best for their patients and are not used to putting the needs or rights of one patient above another. Where child protection is involved, the best course of action for one patient may not be in the best interests of another. This leads to difficulties, and conflicts of interest arise. To which patient should a GP be loyal? The parent or the child? This issue is discussed further in Chapter 6.

Seeing one patient and thinking of another

Normal practice dictates that the patient in front of us is the one about whom we are concerned. However, GPs should remember to consider the risks to children caused by adults with certain medical/social problems (Hobbs *et al.* 1999: 70). When adult patients with drug, alcohol, or mental health problems present in their surgery, GPs need to think, 'Are there children at risk?' Similarly, children living in circumstances where there is domestic violence can be affected in ways that include physical abuse, emotional abuse, and behaviour problems (Hester *et al.* 1998: 44), but the only clue that a child is at risk may be the mother presenting at the surgery with severe bruising or other injuries. Schedule 1 offenders (*see* Chapter 2) also pose risks to children. If a GP is aware that a patient falls into this category and that they have care of, or regular contact with, children, a referral should be made to social services for further assessment.

In all the circumstances described above, there is a need to think if children are at risk on the presentation of adults at consultations, even if the child is not actually present. Doctors are often not alert enough in making the link between the wellbeing of children when only the adult comes to the surgery.

The consequences of 'getting it wrong'

All responsible GPs do their utmost to deliver a high level of clinical care, and as far as possible guard against making mistakes. Referrals to specialists or a local casualty department for second opinions are often made, even though the chance of serious pathology may be slight. If the patient is fine there is relief all round. Although the episode may have caused some anxiety, there is rarely recrimination towards the GP from the patient. Where child protection is concerned, the stakes are different. In some circumstances, the GP may feel that the doctor–patient relationship may be irreparably damaged if a referral is made to social services, especially if further inquiries exonerate the parents. Far from feeling relieved that 'the patient is fine', the parents may distrust their GP, and possibly leave the list. However, the GP has to live with, and may have to answer to, the consequences, if at a later date the child is found to have suffered abuse and a referral was not made.

The model of history, examination, investigation, diagnosis and treatment

The pattern of history, examination, investigation, diagnosis and treatment is followed throughout a doctor's career. However, because of the close interface between medicine and the law, child protection management often does not fit into this sequence, particularly in the management of sexual abuse. For example, a detailed history should not be taken by the doctor when sexual abuse has been suspected or disclosed (evidence may be contaminated by asking the child direct questions), but taken by a specially trained professional – usually a social worker. It is particularly important that a child is not interviewed in the presence of an alleged perpetrator, or someone who may be colluding with a perpetrator (DoH 1999). Nor should GPs undertake detailed examinations when sexual abuse is suspected — these should be carried out by locally designated specialists, who are usually specially trained police surgeons, often in conjunction with community paediatricians or hospital paediatricians (GPs should check their own procedures for local details). It is most important that the examination is carried out once only, to minimise distress to the child. Investigations such as vaginal swabs (for the purpose of proving or disproving sexual abuse) are not taken by the general practitioner but by a police surgeon, so that any results are acceptable in court for evidence purposes. Swabs taken by GPs are not, because the 'evidence trail' cannot be proven. However, should there be a medical need for the GP to examine the child, e.g. bleeding that may need hospital attention, then clearly the GP should carry out an appropriate examination, and instigate any hospital referral that may be necessary (making, of course, a social services referral, as appropriate, also). These are just a few examples when the well-worn pattern of behaviour of GPs is altered — where the referral takes place before the history and examination, which are then carried out by other professionals.

Referral

The need for further investigation of many conditions, specialist treatment or advice leads to referral of a patient for a second opinion to a consultant in the hospital setting — a familiar and frequent component of general practice. Referrals under these circumstances are made with the confidant advice of the GP and the full knowledge and agreement of the patient, and it is unusual for there to be any stress or problem associated with this process. Referrals made to social services are not usually seen in the same relaxed way — there are concerns that once a process has started it cannot be stopped or worries about handling of the situation — and some practitioners and patients alike still see social workers as people who 'come to take children away'. These may be just some of the GP's concerns (*see* Chapter 9). There is also the difference that the referral is outside the medical profession. The GP may feel anxious at having recognised the possibility of abuse and often dreads the next step.

> While professionals should seek, in general, to discuss any concerns with the family and, where possible, seek their agreement to making referrals to social services, *this should only be done where such discussion and agreement-seeking will not place a child at increased risk of significant harm.* (DoH 1999: 40)

It is important that in cases of physical abuse and neglect (*see* below for the position for sexual abuse), practitioners where possible (taking the above situation into account) explain to parents that they are making a referral to social services. Although this may in some cases lead at first to anger, it has been shown that in the long term there is a better outcome from the intervention where parents and professionals can work together in partnership (DoH 1995). An acknowledgement that parents are often under stress when caring for young children can often defuse a situation, and the referral, if handled sensitively, need not damage the doctor–parent relationship. A referral to social services should be seen as another way of accessing help for families. It should also be remembered that in some cases a child may be brought to the practitioner by a parent who hopes that the doctor will recognise something is amiss. It may well be that a referral to social services is exactly what the presenting parent wants but, knowing that the other parent is abusing the child, is not brave enough actually to come out with a reason for bringing the child to the doctor.

In dealing with cases of sexual abuse where, for example, a child discloses such circumstances, detailed consideration should be given as to whether or not parents should be informed of the decision to refer to social services. There may be circumstances where the child would be put at greater risk by discussing the referral before a social worker has had an opportunity to see the child and family. The reasons for this are as follows: firstly the parent may be colluding with the perpetrator (or may be the perpetrator) and if they are then alerted that a referral is being made, there is the risk that pressure will be put on the child to retract his or her statement. Often, the child's statement is the only evidence that sexual abuse has actually occurred. Unlike physical abuse, examination rarely reveals any evidence that sexual abuse has taken place. The only actual evidence may be what the child says and if he or she is frightened into silence, the child is left in a worse position than before and is therefore at greater risk than before revealing what was happening. Secondly, the child may also be physically threatened or actually harmed, because of having 'told'. However, it is important to acknowledge to the child, at a level appropriate with the age and understanding of the child, that you have heard and understood and will arrange help.

It is impossible to cover every clinical circumstance in this text (see Chapter 12 for some case study examples), but, for example, if a parent makes an allegation about another person sexually abusing their child, it is clearly appropriate to explain to the parent that the way forward is to refer to social services. GPs should refer to their local procedures for further guidance.

Further problems may arise if, for example, a teenager discloses to a GP that they are being sexually abused but does not want anybody else to know. This is of course a difficult situation. In general terms, promises of secrecy should not be given and if possible this should be made clear at the beginning of the consultation if it can be foreseen that the consultation will lead to disclosures. However, if a situation arises where a child explains that he or she is being abused before this can be said, it is important to try and convince the child that it is in his or her own best interests that a referral to social services should be made. It is of course possible that the perpetrator may be abusing other children and this also needs to be taken into account in any decision as to whether a referral should be made anyway.

It is difficult to be absolutely prescriptive in these circumstances, but often a patient's understanding and increasing trust over a period of time will lead to consent to contacting social services. A similar situation may also arise if an adult discloses sexual abuse suffered as a child – the same principles apply.

Management is multi-agency and involves several professionals

GPs are used to collaborating with medical colleagues and allied health professionals concerning the management and treatment of their patients. However, when police or social services become involved with patients and require detailed information, many GPs feel distinctly uncomfortable. A regular observation in many child abuse inquiries points to the '... isolation of the GP and the non-involvement in the inter-agency system' (DoH 1991: 13). GPs are naturally concerned about confidentiality issues (*see* Chapter 6), but when a child may be at risk, relevant information should be shared with appropriate professionals (GMC 1995). Lack of trust may limit cross-referral, resulting in poor co-operation (Reder 1993: 66). In order to procure the best interests of the child, a close working relationship between all the professionals involved has to take place. This is at the very heart of child protection management (DoH 1999).

The varying background of the different professionals involved

Each professional involved in managing the child in a child protection case has a slightly different agenda and this can lead to friction unless each understands the other. The doctor–patient relationship is of prime consideration to GPs, and maintaining a good relationship with parents, as well as their children, is seen as very important. The social worker however works entirely by statute (*see* Chapter 9). The welfare of the child is their primary concern. The police are trained to collect evidence and obtain a conviction.

Each profession also uses different jargon and this again can lead to misunderstandings. For example, the words 'significant harm' have a very specific meaning to social workers, whereas to a doctor or lay person the words 'significant harm' merely mean 'important harm', for example. However, 'significant harm' as mentioned in the Children Act has a very distinct connotation (*see* Chapter 2). The medical profession is just as guilty as anyone else of using its own jargon and assuming others understand. GPs need to be aware of using abbreviations in reports, and should explain medical terms.

Use of terminology that the GP does not understand can also cause problems. A social worker might refer to Section 47 during enquiries, but unless the doctor has had specific training, they will not realise that this is part of the Children Act, whereby the social worker has a statutory duty to make enquiries as to the situation of a child and the doctor has an obligation to respond and co-operate.

There are further difficulties when communication between professionals from different disciplines takes place. Beliefs, preconceptions and moral and social standards can hinder effective communication, and '... professional stereotypes and prejudices can colour relations between agencies' (Reder 1993: 66).

Apart from having different backgrounds, training and jargon, the structure of the day of each professional varies. Surgeries, visits and administrative obligations mean that GPs' days are very tightly planned, often with little flexibility. Social workers' days include meetings about their cases, as well as administration, court work, assessments and visits. Often, GPs try to contact a social worker at lunchtime, only to find they are not there. Busy timetables with different priorities can lead to difficulties when one profession tries to contact the other, and can often lead to impatience and antagonism.

Further obstacles in communication across disciplines can also arise if the GP wishes to contact someone senior in, for example, social services, about a specific child. The hospital medical hierarchy, with the consultant ultimately responsible for clinical care, is familiar, but what are the professionals called in the social work ladder? Terms such as line managers, area team managers and district managers are confusing to GPs, and unfortunately the terminology varies from district to district.

Thus it is not surprising, when all the above points are taken into consideration, that professional misunderstandings arise.

Case conferences

Case conferences are frequently the result of the referral to social services of a child who is thought to be at risk. GPs have a low record of attendance for a variety of reasons (Polnay 2000). Even when they do attend, the structure of the conference, its timespan and the way it is managed (Stevenson 1989: 190) are all very different from the type of meeting that a GP is perhaps more used to attending within a primary healthcare team (PHCT). This can lead to misunderstandings and indeed sometimes antagonism between the medical and social work professions. The GP should send a report (see Chapter 7).

Many other professionals have information about the child

When managing a medical problem, information is usually only held in the GP's and, where appropriate, the hospital's notes. The health visitor also has details for her caseload. However, when child protection issues arise, information is held by many others. Up to 72 different professionals can be involved in such cases (Reder 1993: 65)! It is not surprising that each may not be aware of the other's involvement.

The primary healthcare team

Within the primary healthcare team the following have a part to play in child protection:

- Partners of the practice — need to communicate with each other and the rest of the PHCT.

- Locum doctors — must be aware of the practice's system of identifying 'at risk' children.

- Receptionists — they see what goes on in the waiting room or hear what is happening at the end of the telephone.

- Midwife — clearly gains much information about the mother and her new baby.

- Health visitor — probably the most involved (*see* Chapter 8) and is often the linchpin in knowledge of the child and the family.

- Practice nurse — particularly important with regard to new patient registrations and learning about adult patients. Also important in the giving of immunisations to children.

- Practice manager — plays an important part in co-ordination and production of a practice protocol in managing child abuse. The practice manager may also be responsible for keeping child protection procedures up-to-date and organising appropriate training.

- District nurse — may also gain valuable information during visits.

To complicate matters further, much information about a child and his/her family which may be crucial to building up the full picture of the situation may be held by many outside the PHCT, for example:

- social services
- nursery schools
- youth leaders
- casualty departments
- the police
- school teachers
- school nurses
- hospital paediatricians
- community paediatricians
- parents, carers and extended family
- neighbours
- the NSPCC
- home helps
- psychologists
- probation officers.

As the case progresses, solicitors, barristers, magistrates and judges may also become involved.

It is a common scenario that the notes of children who are known to be at risk become thicker and thicker because of the many letters, meetings and conferences that take place about them. There is clearly a problem in co-ordinating information from all these sources.

The child protection register (CPR)

This is described in detail in Chapter 9. Following an initial child protection case conference (ICPC), a child is entered on the child protection register if she/he is believed to be at continuing risk of suffering significant harm. There is no equivalent in medical practice. Although chronic disease registers are kept by practitioners in a computerised or manual system, their purpose is to check that patients are receiving the treatment and monitoring they need. The input is medically based, and the register can only be accessed by practice staff. However the child protection register has input from many sources, and it can be accessed by a variety of appropriate professionals from different disciplines who are concerned about a child's safety. Many GPs are still not used to the process of contacting the child protection register when they are concerned that a child is at risk. However, this is a crucial part of child protection management. The CPR is often the only point of reference that several professionals can key into and it can sometimes provide or collect the crucial missing piece of information that alerts social services, or indeed a GP, that a child is at risk.

Protocols and procedures

Whilst GPs and the medical profession in general are becoming more used to using guidelines and protocols for managing diseases, for example, hypertension, and basing practice on evidence-based medicine, having practice rigidly defined by a document that appears to have its origins in the social services is rather different. The procedures (*see* Chapter 3) originate from the ACPC (*see* Chapter 3) which is a multi-professional committee, and the medical section is usually written with medical collaboration. The basic principles will be the same throughout the country, as the document is based on guidance from *Working Together to Safeguard Children* (DoH 1999), but to complicate matters details may differ from county to county. This again is a different scenario; usually a well-recognised protocol for management is the same wherever the GP is in practice. This could lead to management errors.

Is there one amongst us?

'Bogus doctors' are well documented – those individuals who work their way into the system and practise as doctors but are not medically qualified, perhaps because of a thwarted yearning to be part of the profession. GPs are always advised to be meticulous in checking registration details before employing locums or taking on new partners. A practitioner convicted of improper behaviour with adult patients is a sad but well-documented occurrence. If a colleague seems unfit to practice due to illness, drug or psychiatric problems, the GMC has a recommended route of action to help the doctor and protect the patients (GMC 1993).

However, the presence of a child abuser amongst doctors touches an altogether different nerve. One's natural instinct is not to believe that a colleague could possibly be involved in child abuse. The betrayal of our profession by such people leaves us feeling bewildered and angry. Should there be concern about improper conduct of a colleague with children, the GMC guidance must be followed and appropriate authorities contacted.

The way forward

General practitioners can do much to overcome these difficulties by ensuring that they and their staff have regular training and updating in child protection. Topics to cover should include recognition, how to approach parents when making a referral, procedures, communication issues and local sources of advice. A number of previous enquiry reports have recommended that such programmes be developed (DoH 1991: 33). A successful rolling programme specifically designed for GPs has been developed in Nottingham (Polnay and Blair 1999). Some practices may find helpful *A Safer Practice* (Armstrong 1996), which is a PHCT learning pack. PCG/Ts also have a responsibilty to ensure that they have a mechanism for all staff, including GPs, to be up-to-date in child protection. Additionally, ACPCs usually provide child protection seminars on an inter-agency basis. The British Association for the Study and Prevention of Child Abuse and Neglect (BASPCAN) has branches throughout the country, and organises many seminars on child protection issues, which should be of interest to the GP. There are also varying levels of GP training available, depending on area. Unfortunately, GPs are often reluctant to attend child protection training, probably because of the pressure of many other demands on their time and the relatively low incidence of having to deal with child abuse. However, this low incidence means that it is even more important that training is undertaken regularly, and that GPs know what to do and whom to contact for advice *in advance* of the issue arising. It is too late to discover that crucial phone numbers are missing, or that one is unsure of the correct line of action to take, when the child is in the surgery. The consequences of 'getting it wrong' may be irrevocable.

In addition to training, personal contact with local social workers and the PHCT is helpful in building trust, which in turn helps exchange of information. GPs who have had some training in child protection have an improved attitude towards communication with social workers (Simpson *et al.* 1994).

When all the foregoing factors are considered, it is clear that the GP needs to negotiate many hurdles when managing a child who is at risk of, or has suffered, abuse. Many of these issues are very similar for other professionals involved in child protection, but keeping up-to-date in child protection management and working in co-operation with other agencies is an essential ingredient if the best interests of the child are to be fulfilled.

References

Armstrong H (1996) *A Safer Practice.* The Stationery Office, London.

Department of Health (1991) *Child Abuse. A Study of Inquiry Reports 1980–1989.* HMSO, London.

Department of Health (1995) *Child Protection: Messages from Research.* HMSO, London.

Department of Health (1999) *Working Together to Safeguard Children.* The Stationery Office, London.

General Medical Council (1993) *Professional Conduct and Discipline: Fitness to Practice. Part 4.* General Medical Council, London.

General Medical Council (1995) *Duties of a Doctor.* General Medical Council, London.

Hester M, Pearson C and Harwin N (1998) *Making an Impact. Children and Domestic Violence.* Barnardo's, London.

Hobbs CJ, Hanks HGI and Wynne JM (1999) *Child Abuse and Neglect. A Clinician's Handbook.* Churchill Livingstone, London.

Polnay JC (2000) General practitioners and child protection case conference participation. *Child Abuse Review.* **9**: 108–23.

Polnay JC and Blair M (1999) A model programme for busy learners. *Child Abuse Review.* **8**: 284–8.

Reder P, Duncan S and Gray M (1993) *Beyond Blame.* Routledge, London.

Simpson CM, Simpson RJ, Power KG, Salter A and Williams GJ (1994) GPs and health visitors' participation in child protection case conferences. *Child Abuse Review* **3**: 211–30.

Stevenson O (ed) (1989) *Child Abuse. Public Policy and Professional Practice.* Harvester Wheatsheaf, Hertfordshire.

6
Ethical considerations

Janet Polnay

This has been one of the most difficult areas of child protection to tackle, yet no text on this subject would be complete unless certain issues are addressed. I feel it would be useful to explore from a practitioner's point of view some of the problems that cause particular anxiety in child protection, and indicate sources and principles from which some guidance may be obtained.

GPs generally assume that a child's parent(s) or carer(s) will want the best for their child. They will often have known the family for many years over more than one generation, frequently having parents and their children as patients. However, the interests of abused children and their families may not necessarily coincide. The difficulty in overcoming the psychological barrier in order to make a referral to social services, after the realisation that abuse may be occurring, is not to be underestimated, not least because it can make the GP seem as though they are betraying the adult, who may also be a patient, and therefore breaking trust. It is even more problematic if the diagnosis of abuse is unclear. But the tragic deaths of Jasmine Beckford, Kimberley Carlisle and Tyra Henry indicate that the family environment is not necessarily the safe place for children that has always been thought.

While this chapter does not try to have all the answers to the ethical problems that arise in child protection, GPs' decisions on individual cases may become clearer if certain avenues are discussed and explored.

The United Nations

In 1959 the United Nations issued its first declaration of the rights of children, announcing young people's entitlement to adequate nutrition, free education and medical care (Franklin 1995: 5). Article 19 of the Convention goes on to state that

> State Parties shall take all appropriate ... measures to protect the child from all forms of physical or mental violence, injury or abuse, neglect or negligent treatment ... including sexual abuse, while in the care of parent(s) ... or any other person who has the care of the child. (Human Rights Treaty Series No. 44:7)

The British Government ratified this convention in December 1991, which makes clear all our obligations to children.

Further reference to the Human Rights Bill and how it may affect child protection issues can be found in Chapter 2.

The Children Act 1989

In 1989 the Children Act was passed in Great Britain. This has been described by Lord McKay as, 'the most comprehensive and far-reaching reform of child law which has come before Parliament in living memory' (White et al. 1995: 1) (this quote is from 502 HL official report 5th series, col. 488). The central premises of the Act are, firstly, that the child's welfare is paramount, and, secondly, that parents have responsibilities rather than rights. It emphasises that children are not the possessions of their parents but that children are persons to whom duties are owed (Lyon and Parton 1995: 41).

A further aspect of the Act was the framing of a legal mechanism which opened up the private household so that parental behaviour could become clear, thus making the family more visible to social regulations (Lyon and Parton 1995: 40). This Act is more fully discussed in Chapter 2.

The General Medical Council

> ... make the care of your patient your first concern
> ... respect and protect confidential information (GMC 1995)

In cases of child abuse, the above statements may almost seem contradictory, especially when information on patients who care for children needs to be considered and shared with other professions, such as social services. However, when a child's wellbeing and safety are in question, the child's interests must surely be placed above that of the adult when the following, from *Confidentiality: Protecting and Providing Information* (GMC 2000), is considered:

> If you believe a patient to be a victim of neglect or physical or sexual or emotional abuse, and that the patient cannot give or withold consent to disclosure, you should give information promptly to an appropriate responsible person or statutory agency, where you believe that the disclosure is in the patient's best interests. You should usually inform the patient that you intend to disclose the information before doing so. Such circumstances may arise in relation to children, where concerns about possible abuse need to be shared with other agencies such as social services. Where appropriate you should inform those with parental responsibility about the disclosure. If, for any reason, you believe that the disclosure of information is not in the best interests of an abused or neglected patient, you must still be prepared to justify your decision.

GPs are not used to sharing information with non-medical colleagues. However, the sharing of information is one of the cornerstones in child protection work although in some cases it can be hard to convince doctors to reconcile this issue with the ethics of patient confidentiality. The appropriateness of informing the parents of referral in particular circumstances, especially sexual abuse, has already been discussed in Chapter 5.

Guidance in *Working Together to Safeguard Children* and *Guidelines: Medical Responsibilites*

Working Together to Safeguard Children (DoH 1999) is the Government's guidance for managing child protection and is directed at all professionals who are involved in the care of children. A summary of its contents has been given in Chapter 2. *Child Protection: Medical Responsibilites* (DoH 1995), an addendum to this document, is aimed particularly at members of the medical profession. All GPs should have copies of both these documents in their possession.

The guidance for the medical profession in *Working Together* uses quotes from the 'Confidentiality' section of *Duties of a Doctor* (GMC 1995) and states the position of the medical profession in cases of child protection, emphasising that '... the importance in most circumstances of obtaining a patient's consent to the disclosure of personal information', but makes clear that information may be released to third parties – if necessary without consent – in certain curtain circumstances.

I feel it is worthwhile to quote extensively at this point from the document (DoH 1999):

Disclosure in the patient's medical interests
Problems may arise if you consider that a patient is incapable of giving consent to treatment because of immaturity, illness, or mental incapacity, and you have tried unsuccessfully to persuade the patient to allow an appropriate person to be involved in the consultation. If you are convinced that it is essential in the patient's medical interests, you may disclose

relevant information to an appropriate person or authority. You must tell the patient before disclosing any information. You should remember that the judgement of whether patients are capable of giving or withholding consent to treatment or disclosure must be based on an assessment of their ability to appreciate what the treatment or advice being sought may involve, and not solely on their age. (para. 10).

If you believe a patient to be a victim of neglect or physical or sexual abuse, and unable to give or withhold consent to disclosure, you should usually give this information to an appropriate responsible person or statutory agency, in order to prevent further harm to the patient. In these and similar circumstances, you may release information without the patient's consent, but only if you consider that the patient is unable to give consent, and that the disclosure is in the patient's best medical interests. (para. 11)

Disclosure in the interest of others
Disclosures may be necessary in the public interest where a failure to disclose information may expose the patient, or others, to risk of death or serious harm. In such circumstances you should disclose the information promptly to an appropriate person or authority. (para. 18)

The GMC has confirmed that its guidance on the disclosure of information which may assist in the prevention or detection of abuse, applies both to information about third parties (e.g. adults who may pose a risk of harm to a child), and about children who may be the subject of abuse. (DoH 1999: 82)

I think that it is clear that where children are at risk, appropriate information needs to be shared with the relevant authorities. Furthermore:

Knowledge or belief of abuse and neglect is one of the exceptional circumstances which will usually justify a doctor making disclosure to an appropriate, responsible person or officer of a statutory agency.

The document continues:

The welfare of children must always be regarded as of first importance as their age and vulnerability renders them powerless to protect their own interests ...

All GPs should read the guidance contained in this document (DoH 1995). As in other aspects of medical practice, the course of action depends on the doctor's clinical assessment of the situation in hand.

The child protection procedures

This document is produced by the Area Child Protection Committee of each social services area, and contains local guidance as to the implementation of the Children Act and *Working Together*. The appropriate response to cases of child abuse is described for each professional discipline involved. GPs should be aware of those sections that relate to them, and how their role ties in with the rest of the professions involved in child protection. Its content and role is discussed fully in Chapter 3.

Possible situations where a conflict of interest may occur

Recognition and referral to social services

When abuse is suspected or recognised, a referral to social services must be made. Openness with parents is desirable (except where such discussion may put the child at risk of significant harm; *see* Chapter 5). Where there is doubt as to whether a referral is appropriate, it is helpful to discuss the case with a local professional familiar with child protection issues, such the local designated or named professionals (*see* Chapter 3).

Responding to a Section 47 inquiry

General practitioners are required to respond and co-operate in these inquiries (*see* Chapter 2), which are made when social services believe a child is at risk from or has suffered significant harm. Social workers are required to seek permission of parents '... before discussing a referral about them with other agencies, unless permission seeking may itself place a child at risk from significant harm' (DoH 1999: 41). Also, *see* Chapter 9 for further discussion of this point. Whilst disclosure without consent is a matter for clinical judgement, and doctors need to be prepared to defend their decision (BMA 1996: 58), GPs must balance the risk to the child should there be delay in co-operating with the social worker's inquiry whilst consent is sought.

In cases where a relevant adult has a medical problem (physical or mental) that impinges on the child's safety, GPs need to consider the risk to the child should such information be withheld, but hopefully in most cases consent to release information will already have been obtained by the social worker. The implications for the child's safety would surely be serious indeed should consent be refused.

Case conferences: Reports and attendance

GPs' response nationally to case conferences is poor, whether by report or attendance. Many factors are responsible for this, but confidentiality issues concern some GPs. The *Working Together* document (DoH 1999: 57) emphasises that the case conference record is confidential. The GP's input is also vital, and a report should be submitted if attendance is not possible. It is good practice to submit a report even if the GP does go, to ensure accurate records. If there is relevant information concerning an adult's physical or mental health relating to the child's safety, the BMA advises obtaining the adult's consent (BMA 1996: 89) before release of such information. However, should consent be refused, the implications for the child must be seriously considered. Particularly sensitive information can be given to the chairperson of the conference in private in advance.

Case review (Part 8) and managerial review participation

Paragraph 8.1 of Part 8 of *Working Together* (DoH 1999) states that:

> When a child dies, and abuse or neglect are known or suspected to be a factor in the death, local agencies should consider immediately whether there are other children at risk from harm who need safeguarding ... Thereafter, agencies should consider whether there are any lessons to be learned from the tragedy about the ways in which they work together to safeguard children. Consequently, when a child dies in such circumstances, the ACPC should always conduct a review into the involvement with the child and family of agencies and professionals. Additionally, ACPCs should always consider whether a review should be conducted where a child sustains a potentially life-threatening injury or serious and permanent impairment of health and development, or has been subjected to particularly serious sexual abuse; and the case gives rise to concerns about inter-agency working to protect children.

The aim of the review is that any lessons are learnt and that they are acted on promptly. Social services, the police, hospital medical and nursing staff, health visitors and any other professionals involved with the child and his/her family all have to co-operate in the review process, by allowing the reviewers (senior staff in each organisation) access to their records and by being interviewed about their input to or care of the child and family. GPs are always involved in the care of children, and when the above circumstances arise, will be asked to take part in the review of the 'health' aspect of the child's, and, where relevant, family's, management. This involves a senior medical or nursing colleague (maybe a GP child protection adviser from the local health authority or child protection team member) requesting access to the notes of the index child, siblings, and relevant adults. The GP(s) involved are also interviewed. A report is compiled by each reviewer, which details the chronology of events, action taken, whether the child protection procedures have been followed, and any recommendations. Finally, a sub-committee of the ACPC reads all the reports (which are anonymised), and recommendations made.

Frequently, in these circumstances, the police will rapidly remove the notes from the practice. It is always a good idea to photocopy the notes before releasing them, so that the GP can refer to them again as necessary. The reviewer contacts the GP directly when the notes remain in the practice or gains access to the notes through police contacts if the notes have been possessed.

GPs should '... co-operate with requests for information even where the child's family does not consent' (GMC 2000). Without GP input, the circumstances surrounding the death of the child are incomplete. Crucial information relating to communications between professionals would particularly be missed. Misjudgements, even though only seen in hindsight in a particular case, would be at risk of being repeated in future management if not highlighted, and other professionals need to be made aware of potential pitfalls, by way of recommendations made following the review. Individuals are anonymised before the report is submitted to the Overview Sub-committee.

Inevitably, GPs and other professionals who are subjects of a case review feel anxious that their practice is being scrutinised, but reviewers are sensitive to this and certain procedures, such as sharing the report with the GP concerned before its submission, can go some way to allay anxieties. Much has been learnt from case reviews in the past, and child protection management has been shaped significantly as a result of lessons learnt. Advances can only be made, both for future care of the index family and for children at risk in the future, if all the professionals concerned contribute to these reviews.

A managerial review may be undertaken if there is concern about a child or children, but the criteria for a full case review are not met. In these circumstances, individual agencies and professions organise the process – again GPs' contribution may be crucial to the understanding of the circumstances.

Conclusion

In many aspects of medical practice, answers are not always clear cut and final decisions rest on the clinical judgement of the practitioner. Ethical dilemmas in child protection are no exception. I have endeavoured to guide the reader to some of the principles involved to help with this process. When I have doubts, I consider the following quotations, which may be of help to others when faced with dilemmas in these difficult issues:

> It is important to recognise that it is the child who is the patient to whom the doctor has the primary obligation (Bamford 1996: 672)

and

> ... childhood is a condition of circumstance characterised by powerlessness. (Franklin 1995: 9)

References

Bamford FN (1996) Commentary: A flexible approach – but not too flexible. *BMJ*. **313**: 672.

British Medical Association (1996) *Medical Ethics Today: Its Practice and Philosophy*. BMJ Publishing Group, London.

Department of Health (1995) *Child Protection: Medical Responsibilities*. HMSO, London.

Department of Health (1999) *Working Together to Safeguard Children*. The Stationery Office, London.

Franklin B (1995) The case for children's rights: a progress report. In: Franklin B (ed) *The Handbook of Children's Rights*. Routledge, London.

General Medical Council (1995) *Duties of a Doctor*. General Medical Council, London.

General Medical Council (2000) *Confidentiality: Protecting and Providing Information*. General Medical Council, London.

Lyon C and Parton N (1995) Children's rights and the Children Act 1989. In: Franklin B (ed) *The Handbook of Children's Rights*. Routledge, London.

White R, Carr P and Lowe N (1995) *The Children Act in Practice*. Butterworths, London.

7
The role of the general practitioner

Janet Polnay

The content of this chapter is based on *Working Together to Safeguard Children* (DoH 1999: 19–20) where the GP's role and responsibilities are outlined, recommendations from the Nottinghamshire ACPC arising from lessons learnt following many case reviews (*see* Chapters 1 and 2), and a common sense approach.

Opportunities

The general practitioner is in an ideal position to recognise when a child is potentially at risk. Surgery consultations (by both the child and his/her carers), treatment room sessions, practice baby clinic attendances, family planning opportunities, ante- and post-natal clinics and home visits all help to build up a picture of the child's situation. Information to and from the health visitor, midwife and practice nurse, as well as what receptionists observe in the waiting room or hear on the telephone, can alert the doctor if something is amiss. However, in order for these opportunities to be realised, there are two prerequisites:

- constant awareness that child abuse occurs
- communication between members of the PHCT.

If there is raised awareness, there is increased recognition. Years ago, young children with chronic coughs were given antibiotics as they were thought to have chest infections. When it was realised that they in fact had asthma, the recognition rate of asthma increased, because GPs were more aware of the correct diagnosis, though the actual incidence rate was the same. In a similar way, if the awareness of child abuse presentations is raised, increased recognition will follow. Apart from identifying the different forms of abuse (described in Chapter 11), the psychological barrier of actually accepting that a parent (or carer) can harm a vulnerable child in their charge, has to be overcome.

GPs and the PHCT are also well placed to take part in identifying the 'child in need' (*see* Chapter 9) and should contribute to the assessment of such children and their families when requested to do so (DoH 2000). More emphasis is now being placed on the prevention of abuse following research (DoH 1995). By identifying, assessing and helping those children and families in need, the expectation is that the rates of abuse should fall.

Responsibilities

Staff training

As general practitioners are employers, they are responsible for their staff — for their acts of omission and commission in the carrying out of their duties. GPs need to make sure that receptionists know what to do when they are concerned about a child, and be confident that their practice nurses are fully conversant with the child protection procedures. This is best achieved by ensuring that practice nurses attend regular training courses on child protection issues, which are available locally or nationally. Practice nurses are clearly vital members of the team — often carrying out immunisations, weighing babies at clinic, or dealing with 'minor' injuries in the treatment room. Some practices may find it helpful to invite an outside professional, perhaps from the local Child Protection Advisory Service or ACPC, to come to talk to the practice team and many find it useful for a practice 'child protection protocol' to be compiled. Such a training model has been developed in Nottingham, where a GP experienced, and with a special interest, in child protection visits practices and carries out a training session for the whole practice team.

General practitioner training

As in any other branch of medicine, GPs have a responsibility to keep up-to-date. Local availability of updating sessions vary from one area to another, but every effort should be made to keep abreast of local developments. Whilst there is often a reluctance to attend postgraduate education in this subject, the consequences of error can be far-reaching.

In Nottingham, a locality-based training model has been developed (Polnay and Blair 1999). A community paediatrician and a medical adviser in child protection (with GP experience) teach groups of GPs in local health centres or on practice premises. The sessions emphasise the four points that repeatedly arise as problem areas (for all professionals involved, not just GPs) from enquiries into child deaths or cases of serious public concern (case (Part 8) reviews):

- recognition
- communication
- knowledge of procedures
- note keeping.

Slides and groupwork on case studies are used, and a senior social worker attends some sessions to explain current social services policies, and to act as a resource. This programme, which has been running since 1995, has been highly evaluated by the participants.

Other sources of child protection training should also be accessed (*see* Chapter 5).

Knowledge of ACPC child protection procedures

This is the document that co-ordinates the management of child protection across all professionals that have contact with children (*see* Chapter 3), and is based on government guidance in *Working Together to Safeguard Children* (DoH 1999). It is most important that the procedures are followed meticulously — they will have been drawn up and agreed upon by local senior professionals across disciplines involved in the welfare of children, including the LMC representative, on the ACPC.

It is vital that GPs should be familiar with the local ACPC child protection procedures. The actual format and length of different ACPC procedures varies, but there is usually a section for GPs containing information such as who to contact for advice as well as what action to take when abuse is suspected or recognised. Useful telephone numbers may also be included. These may change from time to time, as can other local policies, e.g. who to telephone for advice — community paediatrician or hospital paediatrician, so it is important that the copy of the procedures in the practice is kept up-to-date.

Communication within the primary healthcare team

Good communication systems are essential in the detection and prevention of child abuse. If opportunities are not to be missed, there must be efficient and easy access for the health visitor to the GP and *vice versa*. Regular meetings, perhaps at the end of a practice baby clinic, should take place, and the health visitor should also have easy access to the GP at other times when necessary. Snatched corridor communications are seldom adequate or safe for the child and family concerned.

Health visitors need to be informed as soon as a child under five years old joins the list, so that a visit can be carried out and the health visiting notes obtained. These often arrive before the GP notes, and may contain vital information, e.g. the child may be on the child protection register. Efficient liaison with school nurses is also essential, so they can be informed when a school age child joins the GP list. The actual mechanisms used to facilitate these channels of communication will vary from one practice to another, but at a basic level a book can be kept of new paediatric patients as they join, which the health visitor and school nurse inspect and sign at frequent and regular intervals. Midwives, district nurses and practice nurses also need to be able to meet with the GP regularly so information can be shared.

Not only do communication systems need to function efficiently, but the nature of relevant information needs to be recognised. Issues such as:

- drug abuse
- domestic violence
- alcohol problems
- mental health problems
- learning difficulties
- schedule 1 offences (*see* Chapter 2)

in parents (or carers) often lead to increased risk for a child. These are situations that may first come to the attention of the GP, but need to be communicated to the health visitor.

The PHCT also needs to be aware that:

- teenage mothers
- single parents
- premature babies

indicate increased risk.

Note tagging

General practitioners have a responsibility to ensure that children on the child protection register (*see* Chapter 9) are easily identifiable by those professionals who care for them, so extra vigilance is possible when these children come to the surgery. Identification can be by computer, a highlighted entry on a summary card in the notes, an extra 'at risk' red card or any other system that suits the practice. However, whichever method is chosen, recognition should be immediately obvious to all members of the PHCT, including locums and GP registrars. Parents are fully aware when children in their care are on the register so this knowledge need not be concealed from them. Some practices may also wish to highlight in the notes incidents that give cause for concern, so that if there are further worrying occurrences (possibly observed by another practitioner) a link can be made. It is also useful to know if a child has had a previous registration. In Nottingham, a red card for insertion in the notes is recommended to note aspects of concern. Increased use of computerisation in general practice can also facilitate recording and cross-referencing of information that gives rise to concern of increased risk.

Siblings' notes

If a child has a sibling on the CPR, this information should be clearly visible in that child's notes. Similarly, a previous unexplained child death in the family should be recorded.

How to identify who is on the child protection register

In some areas, social services may be able to tell individual GPs which of their patients are on the register. The health visitor attached to the practice should also have this information.

Other note keeping requirements

Children (and adults) joining a GP's list should have their notes summarised (if not already done by the previous doctor), so relevant information can be extracted.

Case conference minutes will keep the information up-to-date, and should be filed *with* the appropriate child's notes and *not* separately. Whilst it is recognised that this may be bulky, there is a real danger otherwise that when the child changes GP, the minutes may be left behind. It is also important to record if children are removed from the register.

Ongoing care

GPs clearly have a role in the ongoing care of children – apart from the purely medical aspects. Being aware of family circumstances and the general level of care given to a child can provide valuable information.

Duties

General practitioners have a duty to inform social services when appropriate, that is when they believe a child has suffered significant harm or is at risk of suffering significant harm. The terminology used in the previous sentence is taken from the Children Act 1989 (*see* Chapter 2). The responsibility to refer to social services is made clear in *Working Together to Safeguard Children* (DoH 1999) and in *Confidentiality: Protecting and Providing Information* (GMC 2000) and has been discussed in Chapters 5 and 6.

Persistent parental refusal to take their child to hospital appointments and failure to carry out treatment that a general practitioner has recommended needs to be recognised as neglectful. Failure to take up developmental surveillance – hearing tests etc. – may be because of difficulties such as lack of transport. However, continued lack of uptake of such services for children in the absence of practical considerations is often another example of neglect.

It is expected that GPs communicate their concerns with parents (taking account of the particular circumstances in cases of sexual abuse which may indicate that this action is contra-indicated (see Chapters 5 and 9)), where possible. General practitioners are often worried about doing this, fearing aggression and anger from the parent. However, it should be remembered that sometimes a parent brings a child to the GP in the hope that something will be recognised and action taken. Perhaps the other parent, a step-parent or other person could be abusing the child, and the only way of asking for help is by presenting the child to a doctor. Studies have shown that while there may be anger from the parents when they are informed that a referral to social services is being made, parents would far rather be kept informed from the beginning of concerns than find out later on (DoH 1995).

There is, of course, the risk that a referral will be made to social services and that the concerns will later prove to be unfounded. This is the scenario that every doctor wishes to avoid. There is no easy answer to this dilemma; sometimes we just don't know and have to play safe. It must be remembered that the child's interests are paramount. It is sometimes possible to explain to parents why a referral being made in terms such as: 'I don't understand the explanation, it doesn't seem to add up and I need a second opinion' or 'It is clear you are under stress, and I need to arrange extra help for you.' There are many medical circumstances when GPs ask for second opinions.

In general, parents do realise that professionals have a duty to contact social services when they are concerned about the possibility of child abuse. If handled sensitively, the doctor–patient relationship need not be compromised. It is a risk, but the risk of not contacting social services and missing a case of abuse and the subsequent implications need to be borne in mind.

Responding to social services enquiries under Sections 17 and 47

The above sections of the Children Act have already been explained in Chapter 2. Social workers may need to contact GPs to enquire about a child if they have had a referral from another source (*see* Chapter 9). It is part of the social worker's assessment of a situation to make enquiries from all professionals involved with that child, in order to build up as full a picture as possible of the child and the family circumstances. The GP has a duty to respond to these enquiries. This may, on occasion, involve releasing confidential information about parents or carers of that child. Clearly, this poses ethical and confidentiality issues (*see* Chapter 6).

However, where there is some aspect of the medical history that has a direct bearing on the welfare of the child, and where the child may be at risk if that information is not released, the GP should release that information. The GP clearly would need to check that the person to whom they are talking is a *bona fide* social worker and be reassured that the information is only being used for the wellbeing of the child in question. The GP should document their own actions and why they feel they are justified. There is clearly a difference between detailing the whole of the medical history of the parent to a social worker and only that aspect which is of direct relevance to the child in question.

Case conferences

A GP should be invited to a case conference when it concerns one of their patients. Nationally, GPs' attendance at case conferences has repeatedly been shown to be very poor (Hallet and Birchall 1992: 280). Factors such as not enough notice, poor timing and case conferences lasting too long have been cited as reasons for GPs' non-attendance (Lea-Cox and Hall 1991). More recent work (Polnay 2000) has shown that GPs do not consider attendance at case conferences a priority in their ever-increasing workload. However, GPs should realise the immense importance of their participation in this form.

The height of perfection would be for all GPs to go to all case conferences. Much would be learnt by them about the children for whom they care, as well as the conference providing an opportunity to contribute background knowledge. Clearly, however, this is not possible. A 'next best' is for GPs *always* to submit reports. This has the disadvantage, however, that GPs only offer information that *they* perceive as relevant. For example, negative information, such as not ever having had a consultation with a child, may not seem important to a GP who is asked to give the report, but may be very relevant if the conference is about a child who is severely neglected and underweight. Some areas provide a standard format for GPs to complete for case conferences, which asks for relevant information. However, by not attending, GPs are depriving themselves of the opportunity to learn more about the family. At the very least, a summary of the conference minutes should be carefully filed in the child's and relevant family members' notes, and read whenever possible.

In fact, it is a requirement of *Working Together to Safeguard Children* (DoH 1999) that a written report should be submitted by those professionals who are invited but cannot attend. This is valuable even if it is just to say that they do not know the child very well or that that child has just joined their practice. At the very least, apologies should be sent, either by telephone or in writing, if attendance is not possible. Even if the GP does attend, it is still good practice to submit a report in writing, so that information is recorded accurately.

Co-operating in a case (Part 8) review

Case reviews have been described and explained in Chapters 2 and 6. The conditions under which they take place and the obligation of the GP to contribute have also been discussed. It can be painful and difficult for GPs to take part in this process, which involves a senior GP colleague (or senior nurse or community paediatrician), visiting the practice and scrutinising the notes of the child and any other relevant carer or member of the family or household. The GPs concerned are then interviewed and a report compiled.

The colleague who carries out the case review will do so as sensitively as possible, but the GP may still feel somewhat threatened. However, it is only when all aspects of all the professionals' involvement can be put together, that the pattern of events can be understood. Many lessons have been learnt from these case reviews, and procedures amended over time as a result. The main purpose is not to punish professionals, but to encourage better practice so that vulnerable children are better protected. However, bearing all this in mind, it is clearly in GPs' interests to follow the local child protection procedures carefully, so that, should they become involved in a case review (or managerial review), they have nothing to fear.

Case reviews are often opportunities to improve child protection practice within a partnership. For example, the importance of tagging notes, having regular meetings with the health visitor and keeping copies of referrals are commonly discussed. Also, the importance of a referral being made by the professional who first raises concerns (this may be the GP), rather than relying on another colleague to make the social services referral once the child has been sent to hospital, is an issue frequently addressed. GPs have a duty to co-operate in case reviews, however uncomfortable this may make them feel (GMC 2000).

The practice may undergo further child protection training as a result of a case review. This can involve only GPs and/or can include the whole of the practice, such as receptionists, health visitors, midwives, nursing staff, practice managers and so on. Ultimately, there can be a very positive result with the whole practice working towards protecting children in a much safer way.

Court

In view of the nature of child protection, the GP may be required to appear in court. This can be very stressful. Keeping clear contemporaneous notes and diagrams is essential. The reader is referred to the chapter on courts in *The ABC of Child Abuse* (Mitchels and Meadow 1997) for further information.

This chapter has outlined the opportunities and scope of the GP's responsibilities in child protection – the GP is a key professional, setting the tone for the whole practice, in this important area.

References

Department of Health (1995) *Child Protection: Messages from Research.* HMSO, London.

Department of Health (1999) *Working Together to Safeguard Children.* The Stationery Office, London.

Department of Health (2000) *Framework for the Assessment of Children in Need and their Families.* The Stationery Office, London.

General Medical Council (2000) *Confidentiality: Protecting and Providing Information.* General Medical Council, London.

Hallet C and Birchall E (1992) *Co-ordination and Child Protection: A Review of the Literature.* HMSO, Edinburgh.

Lea-Cox C and Hall A (1991) Attendance of general practitioners at child protection case conferences. *BMJ.* **302**: 1378–9.

Mitchels B and Meadow R (1997) About courts. In: Meadow R (ed) *ABC of Child Abuse* (3e). BMJ Publishing Group, London.

Polnay JC (2000) General practitioners and child protection case conference participation. *Child Abuse Review.* **9**: 108–23.

Polnay JC and Blair M (1999) A model programme for busy learners. *Child Abuse Review.* **8**: 284–8.

8

The role of the health visitor

June Dickens

The scope of health visiting

Health visitors are key contributors to the child protection process. They have a crucial part to play in the promotion of children's health and development and the protection of children from harm. Their unique role in providing a universal, non-stigmatising service gives them privileges that other professionals may not experience, of having access to and regular contact with children and their families. Working closely with GPs and other members of the primary healthcare team (particularly midwives, practice nurses and school nurses), health visitors are well placed to recognise family stresses or circumstances that may lead to abuse or neglect and identify children who have suffered, or who are likely to suffer, significant harm.

Increasingly, health visitors are working with parents caring for children in socially isolated or disadvantaged circumstances. Whilst the majority of these parents wish to, and do, protect and promote the health of their children (often under the most difficult circumstances), research suggests that parents under stress overcome problems more easily when there are sources of family support available. Whatever criticisms have been made of health visiting over the years, it is impossible to deny that they are an excellent resource in terms of local knowledge and linking families with services in the community. These may include baby and child health clinics, self-help/support groups, family centres, play schemes, day care and after school services, to name but a few.

Collaborative working within the primary healthcare team means that there is often an extensive knowledge of family background, which helps in assessing needs and risks. It also enables a significant contribution to be made to child protection conferences and to the long-term support of the child and family.

Clearly, the implementation of PCG/Ts provides real opportunities to review health visiting practice and ensure that skills and expertise are reflected in strategies to meet the needs of the population.

Home visiting, once the cornerstone of health visiting practice, has in many areas been reduced to a birth visit, followed by clinic attendance and client-initiated contact. The Audit Commission Report, *Seen but not Heard* (1995), found that health authorities' attempts to provide a universal healthcare programme to all families have resulted in a failure to provide focused and targeted services for children in need. Recent information from the Department of Health, *Messages From Research* (DoH 1995), suggests that there is a valid argument for targeting resources more effectively and refocusing attention on prevention rather than crisis intervention. This research highlights the need for family support to be offered at an early enough stage, namely at primary level, to prevent child abuse. It also stresses that protection is best achieved by building on the existing strengths of a child's living situation, rather than expecting miracles from isolated and spasmodic interventions. This is especially true in relation to neglect. *Childhood Matters* (National Commission 1997) supports this and stresses that the retention of health visiting as a universal service is vital to the success of child protection strategies.

Assessment is the key to developing strategies to help parents face the challenges of childcare. Structured advice and support can then be offered to assist in the management of situations likely to cause stress. Child-centred interventions may include the development of strategies to cope with crying, feeding, sleeping, toileting or behaviour problems. Adults may need opportunities to talk, to organise their thoughts or to problem-solve, frequently with regard to aspects of their own upbringing, family relationships or the loss of a partner through separation, divorce or bereavement. Individual work offered to adults may include stress management, anger management or strategies to improve self-esteem, assertiveness or social functioning. Research also suggests that providing intervention during the ante-natal period may help to minimise post-natal depression and the subsequent impact on children's behaviour.

Walter Barker (Barker *et al.* 1996) reflects that in the study of 30 000 children whose parents were involved in the Child Development Programme across 24 health authorities, the preceding years since that involvement have seen a reduction by 50% in the level of physical abuse compared with families in the surrounding areas. Parents involved in this programme received regular, home-based, health visiting support and health promotion, either as first-time parents or as a result of assessment demonstrating the need for additional input.

The role of the paediatric liaison health visitor

Despite competing demands on resourcing, many areas have managed to maintain a paediatric liaison health visiting service. Whilst the majority of these posts are managed by community trusts, the work is usually based in hospitals providing paediatric services. Roles and responsibilities are defined locally, although a key component of their work is the facilitation of communication and information sharing between hospital and community health services. Information may necessarily be limited on referral to hospital, with little opportunity for reference to social circumstances or information held by other professionals in the team. Liaison health visitors notify relevant community staff of admissions according to agreed criteria. These may include details of all children under a certain age or those presenting, for

example, as a result of accidents, head injuries, burns or inges-
tions. Similarly, children who have been abused, or for whom
there are concerns, would be reported. This enables colleagues in
the community to contact the hospital to share information,
which assists in the assessment and management of a child's
individual circumstances. A seemingly unremarkable admission
to A&E or hospital may become surprisingly significant when
considered in the context of previous knowledge and experience
shared by colleagues in the community. Another important
aspect of the liaison role is the provision of health visiting
assessment, advice and intervention within the hospital. If a
mother is particularly anxious or is having difficulty with feeding
or other aspects of childcare, support can be given and processes
put in place to ensure that there is continuing care in the
community, which may facilitate early discharge from hospital.

Notification of children attending A&E departments

Revised guidance issued by the Department of Health, *Working
Together to Safeguard Children* (DoH 1999), states that all visits
to A&E should be notified quickly to the child's primary healthcare team and should be recorded in the child's hospital notes.
It is good practice also to notify the health visitor or school
nurse, as appropriate. This alerts staff to the possibility of carers
who seek medical attention from a number of sources in order
to confuse professionals or conceal the repeated nature of a
child's injuries.

Communication and information sharing

Whilst health visitors are said to be part of the primary healthcare team, experience suggests that in many areas this is rhetoric.
There are obviously some excellent examples of true partnership and collaborative working but this is certainly not the

experience of the majority. Studies have shown that multi-disciplinary and multi-agency working frequently mirrors the dysfunctional behaviour exhibited by the families professionals are working with.

Although many practices have regular meetings with health visitors, others do not have a formal arrangement for sharing information and concerns, believing that an 'open door' policy is sufficient. In truth, the latter still sees health visitors hovering outside doors waiting for an opportunity to snatch a quick conversation with a GP in between consultations or at the end of a surgery. This does not promote good team working and provides little opportunity for discussion and planning of joint strategies to support individuals, children and families.

Interestingly, a study in the North of England (Marsh *et al.* 1989) described how GPs perceived themselves as having far better relationships with health visitors than the health visitors saw themselves as having with GPs. On the whole, communication is easier when professionals share the same premises, but current shortages within health visiting establishments means that individuals are now covering caseloads over a wide geographical area which may involve relating to several GP practices.

As thresholds for social work intervention increase, greater responsibility rests with health visitors, nurses and other professionals working with children in the community. Work with children and families where there are concerns about a child's welfare is sensitive and difficult. It creates an enormous amount of stress for individuals, particularly if they feel that they are working in isolation.

Definitions of abuse and thresholds of concern may vary, as do the ways in which information is interpreted and valued. Although government guidance and ACPC procedures are there to inform decision-making and actions, in reality presentations of abuse and neglect are often not so clear-cut. Good practice requires a commitment to joint working, not only with hospital and community colleagues, but also with other agencies.

Effective communication and collaboration are essential within primary healthcare teams if clear messages are to be given to parents or carers about childcare concerns. A health visiting colleague described a disturbing account of poor communication within a team which suggested anxiety or unwillingness on behalf of a GP to become involved in what turned out to be serious non-accidental injury to a four-month-old child. Following a home visit by the GP, the following note arrived on the health visitor's desk: 'Saw Joe today – URTI. Also had what appeared to be finger-tip bruising over ribs? Antibiotics prescribed. I'm away now for two weeks.' The health visitor was placed in a very difficult position. The reference to the bruising needed to be verified, an explanation sought and, as it turned out, a referral made to the social services department. It is difficult for even the most experienced practitioner to enter a house under these circumstances and ask to see marks on a child which the GP had noted but had not discussed with the parents. It does not convey the seriousness of the situation to the parents or give an impression of joint working. In fact this approach is not only dangerous for the child but also likely to cause irreparable damage to working relationships all round.

GPs often worry about expressing concerns to parents, fearing that relationships with the child's carer may be damaged. This appears to be particularly significant where a GP offers care to all members of the family and not just the child. In reality, research suggests that overall, despite their initial distress or anger, parents appreciate openness and honesty, even if it is painful. This approach provides the basis for the development of trust and holds greater credence for future work with families, rather than parents fearing that action will be taken without their knowledge.

Anxiety relating to confidentiality and disclosure of information is not exclusive to GPs. Alison Norman and Christopher Brown (1992) point out that the health visitor's familiarity with families and their emphasis on prevention work may also place them at a disadvantage. They may also have anxieties about jeopardising their relationship with families. The rule of optimism may apply, which makes it very difficult for practitioners to believe that a carer with whom they have been working so closely with can react by deliberately harming their child. The serious nature of the abuse may also be too distressing or awful to contemplate.

Parent-held child health records

The use of parent-held child health records demonstrates a clear commitment on behalf of health professionals to working in partnership with parents and carers. These enable information to be shared in an open and honest way and promote the development of trust in professional and family relationships. Although they provide an excellent medium for sharing information, particularly where care is being offered by several different professionals, reports suggest that, following initial enthusiasm, parents are not producing them consistently and practitioners are not actively encouraging their use. For the majority of children, the records provide essential health information and assist communication; however in respect of child protection concerns, there is great variation in the amount of information recorded. Whilst there is a need for professional judgement and sensitivity in recording, a document which does not indicate that a conference has been held, or that the child's name is on the child protection register (with active social work involvement) and that a multi-agency protection plan is in place, is missing the point and possibly placing the child at even greater risk.

Although it was originally envisaged that there would be no need for supplementary records, it quickly became evident that a personal health record would not provide the means to demonstrate, in full, professional analysis, decision-making and interventions, particularly in relation to children in need and child protection issues.

Notification of children and families moving into and out of the practice

Health visitors and, where appropriate, school nurses need to be informed when families with children register with a general practice. It cannot be assumed that previous records will be forwarded on. As with GP notes, community health records often have difficulty in catching up with families on the move. Whilst it is good practice for health visitors to contact colleagues in a new area when they are aware that a child on the child protection register or a child for whom there are concerns has moved, families frequently leave without informing anyone. Where a forwarding address is known, health visitors are encouraged to make verbal contact with their counterpart covering the address to which the child has moved for the sharing of relevant information. Whilst this is common practice, good practice dictates that the receiving health visitor should also be encouraged to share relevant information with the new GP.

Initial child protection conferences and reviews

Health visitors are regular contributors to child protection conferences, whereas attendance by GPs is, overall, disappointing. Whilst not advocating that this responsibility should be routinely devolved to others, it has to be acknowledged that the growth of PCGs and PCTs will place even more demands on professional time, which is unlikely to improve matters. Where members of the primary healthcare team have had involvement with the child and family, it may be appropriate, depending upon the individual circumstances of the case, to co-ordinate attendance and elect a professional to attend on behalf of the team. Where there are children under five years of age in the family, this would be the health visitor. The team would have to decide whether it would be more appropriate to submit individual reports or compile a joint report for presentation at the conference. The representative would need to discuss issues with relevant colleagues beforehand and have an opportunity subsequently to share the decisions and recommendations of the conference. This information should be clearly documented in all records. Having said this, good practice still dictates that, wherever possible, the GP should attend the conference and, where a medical opinion or contribution is required, there should be no devolving of responsibility on to non-medical staff.

Health visiting role in a protection plan

Following an initial child protection conference, where a decision has been made to enter the name of a child on the child protection register and formulate a protection plan, professionals who will have ongoing involvement with the family will be identified as members of the core group. This will involve the health visitor where there are children under five years of age in the family. Health visitors may be required to monitor the general health of the parents or carers and comment on the quality of the parenting and relationships with the child. They will be expected to assess a child's health, nutrition, growth, development, emotional and physical wellbeing, safety, the impact of their environment and whether the child's basic needs are being met. In these circumstances health visitors need to be clear about the boundaries of their expertise and what services they can realistically offer. Their remit is broad and intervention may include anticipatory and general advice, health promotion, positive parenting advice, or advice about coping mechanisms (management of crying, feeding, sleeping, toileting, behavioural problems). There may also be a need to refer to other sources of help, including the services of voluntary agencies.

The protection plan and the role of the health visitor within that will need to be reviewed regularly in order to assess the effectiveness of interventions. In order to do this the health visitor will need to consider the following questions:

- Is the child safe?

- Have the parents co-operated with the plan?

- Have the interventions brought about positive changes for the child?

- Have the risks to the child reduced?

- Have identified needs been met − if not, why not?

Regular inter-agency reviews will take place to reassess needs and risks, and to evaluate the ongoing protection plan. A decision will then be made as to whether it is appropriate to de-register the child and what level of services would continue to be provided.

Conclusion

With regard to child protection, health visitors' strength lies in prevention. Their work with children and families places them in an ideal position to recognise and act upon signs that a family is under stress or that a child is suffering, or likely to suffer, from significant harm. They are acutely aware of how the health of families and the communities in which they live influences the safety and wellbeing of children. Health visitors have the skills and expertise to meet the new government agenda in promoting positive parenting and supporting children and families in need. In fact, many health visitors would confirm that they are already achieving some of the targets set for their expanded role. They are committed to working together with colleagues from the primary healthcare team and other agencies to improve the quality and accessibility of services for families in order to safeguard children from harm. Communication and collaborative working is the key.

References

Audit Commission Report (1994) *Seen But Not Heard.* HMSO, London.

Barker W (1996) A demotion of professional skills. *Health Visitor.* **10**(69): 407–8.

Department of Health (1995) *Child Protection Messages From Research.* HMSO, London.

Department of Health (1999) *Working Together to Safeguard Children.* The Stationery Office, London.

Marsh GN, Russell D and Russell IT (1989) What do health visitors contribute to the care of children? A study in the north of England. *Journal of the Royal College of General Practitioners.* **39**(322): 201–5.

National Commission of Inquiry into the Prevention of Child Abuse (1997) *Childhood Matters.* The Stationery Office, London.

Norman A and Brown C (1992) In: Cloke C and Naish J (eds) *Key Issues In Child Protection for Health Visitors & Nurses.* Longman Group Ltd, London.

9
The role of social services

John Thorn

The statutory basis of social work

The practice of the majority of professions, and the reasons for that practice, are largely derived from the aggregation of professional experience over time. In other words, the profession itself sets out what should be done, why it should be done and the standard to which it should be done. By contrast, local authority social workers' practice is based, to a very detailed degree, on what the legal statute either requires them to do or allows them to do. There are, of course, social work practice skills, developed from training, research and experience, but any professional judgements or professional procedures must operate within statutory duties and restrictions.

Furthermore, strictly speaking, it is the local authorities who employ social workers through their social services departments who have those statutory duties laid upon them by the law. Social workers act as agents of the local authority and thus, in carrying out their delegated tasks, must follow both their statutory duties and the policies and procedures of their employing authorities. There is also a significant managerial hierarchy within social services departments, and the more important decisions in child protection work will be referred to senior officers. Titles vary from authority to authority but 'team managers', 'service managers' and 'child protection co-ordinators' are common senior posts.

The Children Act 1989 is the legal basis of most children's services social work. There are other Acts that are relevant to specific specialist areas of children's services, such as the Adoption Act, but most of the children's legislation has now been brought together within the framework of the Children Act 1989. This Act is not a particularly thick volume in itself and, of course, all public services have acts of parliament, such as the NHS Acts, Community Care Acts, Education Acts, and Criminal Justice Acts etc., which establish their existence and give a framework for their services. The big difference between the Children Act and these other acts is that the Department of Health published an accompanying set of ten volumes of guidance and regulations to coincide with its introduction and it is these volumes, more than the Act itself, which give the detailed legal directions for social work practice. For example, Volume 1 covers applying for care orders, Volume 2 covers day care provision, Volume 3 covers fostering arrangements and Volume 4 residential care, etc. These volumes of guidance and regulations, were issued by the Secretary of State under Section 7 of the Local Authority Social Services Act 1970, and, as such, although they do not have the full force of statute they 'should be complied with unless local circumstances indicate exceptional reasons which justify a variation'. The force of the word 'should' in legal terms is akin to 'must'.

Working Together to Safeguard Children (DoH 1999), as we have seen in earlier chapters, is the bible of child protection. It too is published as guidance, in the sense described above, by the Secretary of State under the Local Authority Social Services Act 1970 (DoH 1999: viii). Thus, although for all professionals involved with children this document is guidance for best practice, for social workers it defines statutory practice.

The impact of this difference

Care must be taken not to overstate the impact of this difference in the statutory and professional bases of social work and general medical practice, and it is important to acknowledge that primarily the two professions share important values and working partnerships. However, the difference does sometimes present difficulties in practice and it is important to recognise them and work with them.

Perhaps the first and most common issue that arises is over confidentiality. Although the GP has a strong professional ethic about medical confidentiality and would naturally and properly react strongly to any attempt to make him or her breach it, equally the social worker has a legal duty to make enquiries of professionals who know a child and its family when making child protection enquiries, and therefore expects GPs to provide information relevant to those enquiries when asked.

Another common issue is the difference between the flexibility that the doctor enjoys to judge when and how is the best time to tell a patient difficult news, and the legal requirement of a social worker to inform parents of what is happening, however difficult, unless it is not in the child's best interests to do so. This may cause a GP to think of the social service style as very 'confrontational' compared with the 'bedside manner' of good general practice.

A subtle and quite difficult difference can arise over what is best for the child. The social worker has a statutory duty to consider the welfare interests of the child as being 'of paramount importance' and these often conflict with the interests of the parents. However sympathetic to the needs of the parents the social worker may be, this sympathy must be sublimated to their duty to the child. The GP may have both the child and the parents as patients and may be concerned, for example, about the impact of what is happening upon the mental health of a mother. Whereas the GP's professional duties pertain to both the child and mother as patients, the social worker has a paramount duty towards the child enshrined in the law.

What are social services required to do?

Whenever information is brought to the attention of social services which suggests that a child in their area is suffering or is likely to suffer significant harm, or if a child in their area has been taken into police protection, they have a duty to:

- make sufficient enquiries to ascertain whether and to what degree there is a risk to that child
- assess the child's needs
- decide whether and what action is necessary to safeguard and promote the welfare of the child.

Often this package of activity is described as Section 47 enquiries or a Section 47 investigation, after that section of the Children Act 1989 from which the duty arises.

This duty follows from local authorities' general duty to safeguard and promote the welfare of all children in their areas who are deemed to be 'children in need'. These may be children, for example, whose social or educational development is delayed or who have disabilities, and generally any child whose welfare is of concern may be considered to be 'in need'. Such children's needs are assessed and provided for under what are often described as Section 17 duties or Section 17 services, again after the specific section of the Children Act. This includes the duty to provide services to support a child to remain in the care of her or his family unless there are clear indications that it is not in the child's best welfare interests to do so.

Thus it is not simply the case that social services do not have the power to remove a child from the care of its parents without the order of a court; more positively, they have a duty to take steps to keep a child with its parents if at all possible. It is important to note that a child who has been harmed or is at risk of harm is also a 'child in need' in that wider legal sense.

Social workers should apply a systematic approach to the assessment of a child's needs by following the guidance provided in the *Framework for the Assessment of Children in Need and Their Families* (DoH 2000). This framework requires social workers to enquire into and assess the evidence about:

- children's developmental progress:
  - health
  - education
  - emotional and behavioural development
  - identity
  - family and social relationships
  - social presentation
  - self-care skills

- their parents' capacity to respond appropriately to these needs:
  - basic care
  - ensuring safety
  - emotional warmth
  - stimulation
  - guidance and bounds
  - stability

- the wider family and environment context:
  - family history and functioning
  - wider family
  - housing
  - employment
  - income
  - family's social integration
  - community resources.

This framework:

> should provide evidence to help, guide and inform judgements about children's welfare and safety from the first point of contact, through the processes of initial and more detailed core assessments, according to the nature and extent of the child's needs. The provision of appropriate services need not wait until the end of the assessment process, but should be determined according to what is required, and when, to promote the welfare and safety of the child. (DoH 1999: 103)

Providing and co-ordinating services

It will be clear that obtaining the range of evidence necessary to complete what is described in the *Framework for Assessment* requires close co-operation with other agencies, and this is especially the case with child protection work. Social workers will need both to make their own specific contribution and to co-ordinate the contribution of others. Again this is not just a matter of good practice but it is a requirement of the Children Act 1989, both that social services should liaise with other agencies with regard to information and provision of services and that other agencies should co-operate with social services (under Sections 27(1–3) and 47(9–11)) unless it would be unreasonable or prejudicial to their services to do so.

In carrying out the enquiries/investigation which follow receipt of a child protection referral, the social services will normally check their own records and health, education, and police records, and those of any other agencies known to have some involvement with the child. This is because they are not simply concerned with the immediate incident, such as a small child being bruised or left alone by a parent, but also about the context of the incident, how it may relate to what is already known about the child and her or his family and whether the incident is part of a pattern that might give it greater or lesser significance.

Within 24 hours of receipt of a referral expressing concerns about a child's welfare, social workers should decide whether there are concerns about the child's health and development, or actual and/or potential harm which justify further enquiries, assessment or intervention. Referrals may lead to no further action, directly to the provision of services or other help – including that from other agencies – and/or to a fuller initial assessment of the needs and circumstances of the child, which may, in turn, be followed by Section 47 enquiries. Any initial assessment should be completed within seven working days of the date of referral but it may be much briefer if it becomes apparent that the criteria for Section 47 enquiries are met.

Social workers should seek parents' permission before discussing a referral about them with other agencies, *unless permission seeking may itself place a child at risk of significant harm.* This is a difficult area since there may be practical as well as policy reasons why it is not appropriate to obtain a subject's permission before discussing him or her with other agencies. For example, it has become common practice in cases of suspected sexual abuse not to inform parents that enquiries are being made until a clear set of professional concerns has been brought together by sharing information. This is because of the difficulties in obtaining forensic evidence and the importance of the child's verbal evidence following the coming together of these professional concerns. If parents are informed too early, they may threaten the child and prevent him or her from speaking about what has happened. These sorts of consideration should be explained by social workers to help other professionals to decide what information they should provide in the absence of parents' permission (*see also* Chapter 5).

In many cases, particularly those concerning small children or sexual allegations, social services will work closely with the police from the outset of their enquiries because of the helpfulness of the investigative skills that police officers have and the fact that the police themselves may have professional concerns about whether criminal offences, such as assault or child cruelty, have been committed. In some cases a medical examination will be crucial to explaining how serious an injury may be and how it may have occurred and, of course, as a preliminary to appropriate medical treatment. Whenever the enquiries move from the initial to the Section 47 stage there should be a strategy discussion between social services, the police and any other professional groups who might be involved in progressing the enquires. This may happen at a meeting but may, in urgent cases, be by telephone – particularly if there is a need to take immediate action to secure the safety of a child.

Social workers working alongside police officers will follow the *Memorandum of Good Practice* (DoH, Home Office 1992)

which provides detailed practice guidance with regard to inter-
viewing child witnesses, especially in circumstances where it
is necessary to record their interviews on videotape. A number
of specialist social workers and police officers have undertaken
specific training on videotape interview practice.

The child protection register

An important enquiry that social services will always make
is of the child protection register. This is an important inter-
agency tool which, although usually managed by the social
services department, is accessible by all professionals involved
with children. Most registers contain not simply a list of children who are currently considered to be at risk, but also records
of children who have previously been on the register, also siblings and adults (abusing adults often move between partners
and thus enter new families) and, most importantly, they keep
records of previous register enquiries. Thus a social worker
checking the register may find, for example, that although the
child they are concerned with is not on the register, there have
been previous register checks on that child in the past three
months from a teacher and a health visitor who had no specific
referral to make but were concerned enough to want to know
whether the child was on the register. The social worker would
quickly contact that teacher and health visitor to enquire about
those concerns. Most registers have a protocol where a referral
is triggered if a certain number of register checks are made.

The initial child protection conference

The social services' co-ordinating role is very prominent at
the initial child protection conference, where all of the professionals who have involvement with the child and the family are
brought together and the information that has been gathered in

the course of the enquiries is considered. The parents will also attend this conference unless there are good reasons otherwise. A final assessment is made of the significance of the risk to the child and what the child's protection needs are, and a decision is made as to whether a child protection plan is necessary and thus whether the child's name should be placed on the child protection register.

This conference should be held within 15 working days of the strategy discussion which led to the Section 47 enquiries. The Chair of the conference will usually be a senior social services officer, but the decision-making process for conferences may vary from area to area according to the local Area Child Protection Committee procedures. In some areas the professionals attending the conference formally vote on whether the child's name should be placed on the child protection register, whereas in others the decision is an executive decision of the Chair based upon a consideration of the views and advice of the members of the conference. In either case, the registration decision and its consequences are a matter on which social services must take a lead but cannot effectively deal with alone.

Inter-agency contributions and consensus are the keys to effective child protection work. Good decisions have to be informed decisions and sometimes the information that one agency or professional has makes more sense in the light of, or perhaps throws light upon, the information that another professional contributes in a conference. The role of the social services is to bring that otherwise disconnected information together. Likewise, the judgement about the degree of harm or risk to a child is often multi-faceted and is not simply a social work one. For example, a doctor will have professional judgement about the immediate and long-term harm of a particular injury, a teacher will have a judgement about the potential harm of the educational delay presented by a child, a health visitor will have a judgement about the emotional harm of a mother's poor bonding with her child, a social worker will have judgement about the harm being caused by a child's isolated position within a sibling group, etc. The Chair's role is to bring all of those professionals' perspectives on the risk to the child together to form a judgement about overall risk.

What is risk?

In many child protection cases, the significance of an injury, how it was caused and who caused it are all clear and it is a relatively easy task to make a judgement about harm and what is needed to protect a child from harm. In many other cases, matters are far from being that clear. For example, cases where there has been an injury but neither parent will admit to having caused it, or even to knowing how it may have been caused, are quite common. Even cases where there have been deaths to previous children in suspicious circumstances, but not clear proof of the cause, occur uncomfortably regularly. It is very difficult to assess risk in such circumstances, but that is social services' task. It does occasionally lead to professional disagreements in circumstances such as, for example, when a child's name is placed on a child protection register because there are worrying signs, but no clear 'proof', that a sibling's 'cot death' was caused by a parent, especially when there is a lot of natural sympathy for the rather inadequate parents at whom the finger of blame is pointed by such a decision.

In determining 'risk', the classic risk assessment model suggests that the degree of risk is a factor in both the likelihood of the harm happening and the seriousness of the harm *should* it happen. Thus a 90% chance of sustaining a minor bruise is a much smaller 'risk' than a 5% chance of sustaining death, even though it is 18 times more likely. Thus in determining decisions in child protection cases, great care must be taken not to confuse risk with the simpler question of how far it can be proved that a parent did or did not harm their child.

The other often controversial aspect of child protection decisions is that they are rarely risk-free. Social services know well, for example, that decisions to remove children from their parents are probably some of the most risky decisions to make. The emotional trauma for a child of being separated from his or her primary carer, the ensuing protracted legal proceedings and contact arrangements, the difficulties of placing sibling groups together in foster care, etc., are all known to be potentially very harmful to a child.

The child protection plan

The purpose of placing a child's name on the child protection register is to ensure that there is an effective plan to protect the child. Again, social services have a duty to ensure that such plans exist and that the protective services of the 'core group' of professionals involved with the child are co-ordinated by a social worker acting as a 'keyworker'.

Social services may offer a range of services, including case-work or counselling for parents or children, day care or parenting skills training at a family centre, domestic help in the home and foster care on a temporary basis. Other professions will offer crucial complementary services. Primary healthcare teams are nearly always involved in the core groups and child protection plans for younger children in particular, where child health surveillance and health visiting play a vital role.

It will be observed that the sorts of service briefly described above are not specific to child protection – they would also be offered to other children and other parents with needs for social and medical support. This is indicative of the important debate, raised by the Department of Health's *Messages from Research* (DoH 1995), about how far such services should be delivered within a child protection framework when they could be delivered within a general family support framework, particularly when parents are co-operative, since, as has been noted earlier, children who need protective services are also 'children in need' in the wider legal sense. Social services departments are keen to provide family support and preventative measures when these can avoid the necessity for child protection action. Why, then, invoke the heavy and stigmatic panoply of child protection when social services can deliver and co-ordinate inter-agency services under Section 17 of the Children Act?

The answer is simple in principle but taxing in practice. It is a matter of *the significance of the harm and the degree of risk*. It is not just whether parents are co-operative, though that is an important factor, because many inadequate parents try hard to be co-operative and evidently care very much about their children, but their lack of parenting skills place their children at significant risk. There are circumstances in which, although the parents are co-operating, the significance of the risk needs to identified very clearly, for both the parents and the professionals working with them, and services need to be delivered and co-ordinated in a way that keeps that risk at the forefront of everyone's mind in a child-focused way.

Conclusion

In summary, a social services department is the essential participant in child protection work, not only because it has the statutory duty to investigate, assess need and deliver its own protective services to children at risk of significant harm, but also because it has the statutory duty to obtain and co-ordinate the services of other public service professionals where this will assist in protecting such children. It is legally the lead agency, but very much the leader of a partnership of professionals whose services complement one another to provide effective child protection. Social workers have specific training and experience in child protection work, not just in terms of intervention with the child and family, but also in facilitating the inter-agency system, which is key to best practice.

There is a public fear of child protection services and, as we have indicated, an ongoing debate about how far it is necessary to invoke the child protection framework when other family support frameworks are available. However, it is important to emphasise that child protection services are not rollercoasters, which are impossible to stop once started, and they are certainly not as draconian as the public often fear. The Department of Health's research (DoH 1995: 28) indicated that in 1992, of 160 000 child protection enquiries initiated, only 24 500 resulted in the children's names being placed on the child protection register, and only 3000 children were removed from their parents' care. The fact that such a relatively large number of enquiries resulted in such a relatively small number of removals is open to considerable interpretation, hence the debate, but it does suggest that the most serious action is not taken lightly and only occurs after the most careful consideration.

References

Department of Health, Home Office (1992) *Memorandum of Good Practice on Video Recorded Interviews with Child Witnesses for Criminal Proceedings.* HMSO, London.

Department of Health (1995) *Child Protection: Messages from Research.* HMSO, London.

Department of Health (1999) *Working Together to Safeguard Children.* The Stationery Office, London.

Department of Health (2000) *Framework for the Assessment of Children in Need and Their Families.* The Stationery Office, London.

10
Police involvement in child protection

Michael Page

Protecting life and preventing crime are primary tasks of the police. Children are citizens who have the right to the protection offered by the criminal law. The police have a duty and responsibility to investigate criminal offences committed against children, and such investigations should be carried out sensitively, thoroughly and professionally.

Working Together to Safeguard Children (DoH 1999)

Aim of the chapter

The aim of this chapter is to explain the role and duties of the police in child protection and to address the principal fears expressed by general practitioners with regard to that involvement. The four main fears seem to be:

- that the police investigation will not be conducted sensitively
- that doctor–patient confidentiality will be breached
- that they will have to attend court as a prosecution witness
- that they will be initiating something over which they can have no control afterwards.

Why the police are involved in child protection

The police are integral to the multi-agency responsibility for the protection of children, a factor acknowledged in the quote from *Working Together to Safeguard Children* (DoH 1999) included above. What they bring is their experience of conducting investigations to the high standard of proof demanded by criminal law.

In all areas of England and Wales, Area Child Protection Committees (*see* Chapter 3) formulate local policy and the police feature strongly in this joint agency approach to the protection of children. It is a misconception that their involvement in an investigation is with the simple objective of securing the conviction of a suspected offender; it is actually with a much broader objective of participating in a multi-agency enquiry to establish the facts of a situation with the ultimate aim of ensuring a child is protected. Indeed, evidence gathered in interviews involving the police might subsequently only be used in civil proceedings instigated by another agency for the protection of the child.

The police have officers specially trained for this role. In fact, in most areas there are dedicated units for dealing with abused children and other vulnerable witnesses, and they are acknowledged as having high levels of skill in this work. In addition, the police possess emergency powers for the protection of children not held by other agencies.

Parental responsibility and the police

Parental responsibility within the terms of the Children Act 1989, means the child's:

- natural mother
- natural father if the child's parents were married at the time of the child's birth

- natural father if a parental responsibility agreement has been drawn up in the form prescribed by the Lord Chancellor

- any person having parental responsibility by virtue of some form of court order (Sections 2 and 4 of the Children Act 1989).

See Chapter 2 for further details on parental responsibility and the decision contained within the Lord Chancellor's Department Consultation Paper (1998) concerning compatibility with the Human Rights Act.

It is important to note that the use of police protection does *not* give police officers parental responsibility. This is particularly notable regarding consent to medical examinations.

The emergency powers of the police

In order to fulfil the often urgent need to protect people, the police are given a variety of powers. For example, they have power under the Police and Criminal Evidence Act 1984, Section 17(1e) to enter premises without a warrant in order to save life or limb. This power does not necessarily authorise the removal of children from those premises, but where a constable believes a child is likely to suffer 'significant harm' (explained in Chapter 2) there is a power to then take that child into 'police protection' for up to 72 hours without a court order. (All police officers, regardless of rank, hold the office of 'constable'.)

Police protection

Under Section 46 of the Children Act 1989, a constable who has reasonable cause to believe that a child would otherwise be likely to suffer significant harm may:

- remove a child to suitable accommodation and keep her or him there

- take such steps as are reasonable to ensure that the child's removal from any hospital, or other place in which she or he is then being accommodated, is prevented.

A child in respect of whom this power has been exercised is referred to as having been taken into *police protection* (totally separate from, and not to be confused with, the emergency protection orders explained in Chapter 2).

As soon as practicable after taking a child into police protection, the constable concerned must do the following.

- Inform the local authority, within whose area the child was found, of the steps that have been, and are proposed to be, taken with respect to the child, and the reasons for taking them.

- Give details to the authority within whose area the child is ordinarily resident (referred to as the 'appropriate authority') of the place at which the child is being accommodated.

- Inform the child (if she or he appears capable of understanding):
  − of the steps that have been taken with respect to her or him under this Section and of the reasons for taking them
  − of the further steps that may be taken with respect to her or him under this Section.

- Take such steps as are reasonably practicable to discover the wishes and feelings of the child.

- Ensure that the case is inquired into by a *designated officer* (this is someone not involved in the inquiry and often, although not always, of the rank of Inspector) nominated for the purposes of this section by the Chief Officer of Police for the area concerned.

- In cases in which the child was taken into police protection and taken to accommodation not provided *either*:
  - by or on behalf of a local authority *or*
  - as a refuge in compliance with the requirements of Section 51 of the Children Act

  the constable must ensure that she or he is moved to accommodation that is provided as above.

The constable is also required, as soon as is reasonably practicable after taking a child into police protection, to take such steps as are reasonably practicable to inform:

- the child's parents

- every person who is not a parent of hers or his but who has parental responsibility for her or him

- any other person with whom the child was living immediately before being taken into police protection.

They must be informed of the steps taken by the constable in respect of the child, the reason for taking them and the further steps proposed to be taken under this section.

The designated officer has statutory duties independent of those of the constable. He or she must enquire into the case and, on completion of that enquiry, must release the child from police protection unless there is still reasonable cause to believe that the child would be likely to suffer significant harm if so released.

In any case, no child can be kept in police protection for more than 72 hours. The designated officer may, where appropriate, apply for an emergency protection order (EPO) (*see* Chapter 2). This is whether or not the local authority agrees to it or is aware of it, although the guidance is that good inter-agency communication should mean the police never find themselves in this position.

It is not possible to extend police-initiated emergency protection orders. The maximum period of police-instigated protection under an EPO is eight days. The local authority must be involved in seeking further protection should it be necessary.

Whilst a child is being kept in police protection:

- Neither the constable concerned nor the designated officer shall have parental responsibility for her or him.

- The designated officer shall do all that is reasonable in the circumstances for the purpose of safeguarding or promoting the child's welfare (having regard in particular to the length of time for which the child will be so protected).

- The designated officer, if he or she believes it to be appropriate, reasonable and in the child's best interests, shall allow contact with:
  - the child's parents
  - any person who is not a parent of the child but who has parental responsibility for that child
  - any person with whom that child was living immediately before she or he was taken into police protection
  - any person in whose favour a contact order is in force with respect to the child
  - any person who is allowed to have contact with the child by virtue of an order under Section 34 of the Act (parental contact etc. with children in care)
  - any person acting on behalf of any of those persons.

It is perhaps worth repeating that, although a child might be under police protection and a designated officer will have statutory responsibilities for the period of that protection, the child will be not be accommodated on police premises. In almost all cases, the child will be cared for on health or social services premises.

The use of the powers

Although a child can be held in police protection for up to 72 hours without legal challenge, it is a considerable reduction of what was allowed under previous legislation and is in keeping with the general policy to restrict the length of operation of emergency powers. The aim is to ensure that no child taken into police protection need be accommodated in a police station and that his or her reception into local authority accommodation is achieved with the minimum of trauma.

This is a power that is exercised sparingly but comes into its own when, for example, parents attempt to remove children from hospitals or indeed, surgeries. In fact, only the police can take the urgent action required when a child is presented at a surgery with injuries suspected to be as a result of abuse and there are fears for the child's safety because the parent is insisting on taking the child away.

The *raison d'être* of these powers is to enable an instant response to such a situation without recourse to a court. Even so, there is still a requirement for the police to then liaise with local authorities as soon as is practicable concerning the accommodation of the child.

It is against this background of inter-agency co-operation and multi-agency involvement in strategy decisions and case conferences, that the police conduct their investigations. Specialist officers usually conduct them and this is done discreetly, correctly and jointly. In common with all agencies, the welfare and protection of the child is the primary aim of the police.

Working together with other agencies

The principal of 'working together' was established following recommendations contained in the Cleveland Report (DHSS 1988).

The guidance for inter-agency co-operation is now contained in the document *Working Together to Safeguard Children* and it includes sections for the police and, indeed, for GPs (DoH 1999). But more detailed guidance is usually contained in the local Area Child Protection Committee's procedures.

No single agency or individual can work alone; professionals working together and sharing information is more than an expectation, it is a duty.

Breaching confidentiality

In the matter of confidentiality, it would be wrong to assume that a GP cannot or should not disclose any information to the police. Confidentiality is not absolute in medicine.

The General Medical Council have produced guidance on this issue (GMC 1995), which is reinforced in Section 7:39 of the document *Working Together to Safeguard Children* (DoH 1999). They emphasise the importance, in most circumstances, of obtaining the patient's consent to the disclosure, but make the point that information may be released to third parties without that consent in certain instances, particularly if the welfare of a child is at risk as a result (*see* Chapter 6).

It is also worth pointing out that, unless there is a good reason for not doing so, the police may often have sought permission from the patient for access to records before approaching the GP.

Through Area Child Protection Committees, there are local agreements about joint working and sharing of information (to some measure, this is being extended to cover vulnerable adults too). A key principle is that the protection of children is paramount to all the member agencies of those committees. It is usually in accordance with these agreements that the police make their request for information.

As a last resort, there is of course the power for a judge to make an order for medical information in the case of serious arrestable offences. Serious assault of a child would normally fall into that category.

Recording evidence

Quite obviously, the GP and other members of the primary healthcare team are in a key position to identify a child who is in need of protection and will gather evidence as part of their normal role. It is therefore imperative to ensure that there are strategies within the practice for ensuring concerns are brought to the attention of the GP and that the evidence gathered is of the highest integrity.

In order to ensure this and to reduce the risk of challenge in the future, good record keeping is essential whenever there are grounds for suspecting abuse may be a factor in the life of a child patient or that of his/her siblings. This may not, of course, be presented in the most obvious way but may, for example, be as a result of domestic violence being an issue within a family. Whatever the grounds for suspicion, the need to keep accurate records is essential and the following is offered as guidance:

- **All notes should be made contemporaneously** and should be as comprehensive as possible. Doctors will obviously need to be aware of the right of patients to access medical records and reports and also of the fact that they may later be required in court. Recording the time and date of making the notes is particularly helpful in averting challenges as to their accuracy later. This applies equally to paperless notes. The trial of Dr Harold Shipman demonstrated how computer entries can be the subject of an audit trail showing when entries were generated or altered.

- **Use accurate terminology**. There may be a considerable lapse of time before information from records is required and precise terminology, e.g. calling a cut a cut and not a laceration, not only provides better evidence, but may also avoid difficult questions or challenges in a witness box at a later date.

- **Do not leave gaps in notes**. This avoids any allegation that spaces were used for making entries later; another issue highlighted in the Shipman trial.

- **Record only facts**. Avoid judgements, speculation and opinion that cannot be substantiated.

- **Record actual words used**, if a child discloses information of abuse. Date and time the entry, record your own responses and questions accurately and be conscious of the need not to ask more questions than are necessary at the time. A formal interview will probably be conducted later by those charged with that task and the number of occasions when a child has to relive events should be kept to a minimum.

- **Keep a copy** of any notes given to the police, for future reference.

- **Ensure that all records are kept together**. This includes not only the patient's medical record but all other relevant documents, e.g. body maps, referral letters and details of discussions with and requests for information from other agencies. Where police and/or social services enquiries do not result in the substantiation of a referral, the records still may be required in the future for such enquiries. It is therefore imperative that the records are kept carefully.

- **Accurate completion of forms is essential**. In a crown court case recently, a doctor endured some very difficult questioning after stating on a form that a high vaginal swab had been taken from a four-year-old child when in fact it was a vulval swab that had been obtained.

If there is a prosecution, the police, in conformity with the Criminal Procedure and Investigations Act 1996, will always have disclosed the existence of records, and a judge can require their production. It necessarily follows that their author may be called as a witness, but if the records have been made in accordance with the guidance offered, the opportunities for challenge should be reduced, as should the stress for the witness.

Where the enquiry relates to a child death, medical records automatically become the property of the Coroner, but a police officer acting on the Coroner's behalf will usually make the request for them.

Child protection conferences

The police have an obligation to attend initial child protection conferences and will usually submit a written report and attend. In many cases, the officer attending will have been involved in the enquiry, although this can vary according to local policy or circumstances.

The best way for a GP to retain influence and maintain involvement after a referral has been made is to participate in the child protection conference process. (Child protection conferences are explained in detail in Chapter 9.)

Conclusion

Over recent years, a great deal of knowledge and skill has been developed in the field of child protection and the police have no lesser part to play in this than social services, GPs or, indeed, any other of the relevant agencies. It is imperative that all agencies participate fully, discreetly and professionally, not simply because failure to do so could lead to disciplinary action and/or claims for negligence, but because it is in the best interests of our children to do so.

References

Department of Health (1999) *Working Together to Safeguard Children*. The Stationery Office, London.

Department of Health and Social Security (1988) *Report of the Committee of Inquiry into Child Abuse in Cleveland*. HMSO, London.

General Medical Council (1995) *Confidentiality*. General Medical Council, London.

Home Office (1984) *Police and Criminal Evidence Act*. HMSO, London.

Home Office (1989) *Children Act*. HMSO, London.

Home Office (1996) *Criminal Procedure and Investigations Act*. HMSO, London.

11
Recognition of child abuse

Yin Ng

Definitions

The following definitions are used both in *Working Together to Safeguard Children* (DoH 1999) and for the purpose of registration on the child protection register. It must be remembered that a child may suffer more than one type of abuse.

Physical abuse

Physical abuse may involve hitting, shaking, throwing, poisoning, burning, scalding, drowning, suffocating, or otherwise causing physical harm to a child. Munchausen Syndrome by Proxy may also constitute physical abuse, whereby a parent or carer feigns the symptoms of, or deliberately causes, ill health in a child.

Emotional abuse

Emotional abuse is the persistent emotional ill-treatment of a child such as to cause severe and persistent adverse effects on the child's emotional development. It may involve conveying to children that they are worthless or unloved, inadequate, or valued only insofar as they meet the needs of another person.

It may involve causing children frequently to feel frightened or in danger, or the exploitation or corruption of children. Some level of emotional abuse is involved in all types of ill-treatment of a child, though it may also occur on its own.

Neglect

Neglect is the persistent failure to meet a child's basic physical and psychological needs, possibly resulting in the serious impairment of the child's health or development. It may involve a parent or carer failing to provide adequate food, shelter and clothing, failing to protect a child from physical harm or danger, or the failure to ensure access to appropriate medical care or treatment. It may also include neglect of a child's basic emotional needs.

Sexual abuse

Sexual abuse involves forcing or enticing a child or young person to take part in sexual activities, whether or not the child is aware of what is happening. The activities may involve physical contact, including penetrative or non-penetrative acts. They may include non-contact activities, such as involving children in looking at pornographic material or watching sexual activities, or encouraging children to behave in sexually inappropriate ways.

Presentation

An allegation of child abuse may be presented to you by the child/young person, by a parent/carer or by a social worker, a police officer or the NSPCC (these are the statutory agencies). Alternatively, the possibility may occur to you because of the combination of symptoms and signs.

The general principles of clinical assessment apply in these situations. Taking a careful history, performing an appropriate examination and recording your findings are essential (*see* Chapter 5 for the special considerations for sexual abuse). Awareness of your local child protection procedures is also essential.

In some cases, the diagnosis or disclosure is clear and your plan of action is obvious. In other cases, discussion with colleagues in the primary healthcare team, other professionals involved with the child/family and with social services will be needed before a decision is made that an abusive situation exists. Remember that identification of abuse can be difficult and usually both social and medical assessment are needed.

Characteristic features in the history and examination

This section outlines some of the symptoms and signs of child abuse. Some of these features on their own should alert the clinician to the possibility of child abuse. However it must also be remembered that sometimes there may be an innocent explanation for the findings and it is therefore important for as thorough and sensitive an assessment as possible.

General

- Delay in presentation/seeking medical advice.

- Changing accounts are given, or these are vague and lacking in detail.

- History is not consistent with findings on examination.

- Injury is not consistent with the child's developmental level — particularly relevant if the child is very young or if the child is disabled.

- History of shaking, especially of a baby, must be taken seriously. Significant forces similar to those generated by whiplash trauma may be produced, resulting in serious head and chest or abdominal injuries.

- Inappropriate responses from parents or carers. For example, a parent may seem unconcerned about a serious injury.

- Unrealistic expectations/perceptions of parents/carers. For example, a parent may blame the child for causing the injury even when it is apparent that the child is developmentally not yet able to do so.

- Child's interactions with parents/carers, particularly 'frozen watchfulness', wariness or fear, or seeming sad. Frozen watchfulness is a late sign and results from repeated physical and emotional abuse over a period of time.

- What the child says has happened, if she/he is old enough to be seen on their own.

- Unusual site of injury without a consistent history e.g. behind the ear, in the hair, in the mouth, soft tissue areas such as the buttocks. It is important to remember to look for injuries in those areas of the body that are usually hidden from easy view. It is well recognised that perpetrators of physical abuse often mark children on parts of the body that are not so visible.

- Extensive bruising – there may be a medical cause for this, such as a bleeding disorder. In cases where there is no medical explanation found, a thorough social work assessment must be done.

- Many bruises/scars of different ages: Is this an accident-prone child? Is there a medical problem, e.g. of balance, which is causing these incidents? Is there a lack of parental care?

- Unexplained injury/illness, particularly if there is a recurrent pattern of this occurring. The GP records and/or GP's knowledge may be important in identifying such situations.

- Previous suspicions or record of abuse, or a history of multi-generational abuse. The GP records and/or knowledge may be crucial. The importance of making a child protection register enquiry cannot be over-emphasised.

- Indications of or previous history of domestic violence. The GP's knowledge of the family and that of other members of the primary healthcare team is important in raising awareness that children may be harmed in these situations. There is increasing evidence that children who witness and experience such violence have a high risk of suffering emotional harm, even if they are not physically injured.

- The GP's knowledge of the family situation. This important point has been mentioned earlier in this section and cannot be over-emphasised. For example, the GP may be the only professional who has knowledge of the mental health difficulties of a parent/carer and is therefore the only one who can judge how likely these are to affect his/her ability to look after the children in their care safely.

It must be remembered that a child may suffer from different types of abuse at the same time, and that a child with a genuine medical condition or disability may also suffer abuse.

More specific characteristics

Physical abuse

Bruises

- Facial bruising and/or other injuries in a non-mobile child such as a very young baby.

- Bruising or other injuries in or around the mouth, including the frenulum, particularly in young babies. A torn frenulum may be caused accidentally, but there is usually a good description given of an accident and immediate help is usually sought. A healed tear of the frenulum will persist and its presence could indicate previous abuse.

- Grasp marks on limbs or fingertip bruising on the chest of a small child.

- Bruising or other injuries to unusual sites for accidental injury or to sites which may be hidden from normal view, e.g. behind or on the ear, back, abdomen, buttocks, head, neck, face, genital area.

- Outline bruising, e.g. hand prints, shoe marks, belt marks.

- Extent or type of bruising is not consistent with history given, e.g. both eyes are bruised with no history given of forceful knock to head.

- Differential diagnoses – clotting/bleeding disorders, birth-marks, skin disorders.

Burns and scalds

- Sites of injury – face and head, perineum, buttocks and genitalia, the hands (often the dorsal surface), the feet (may be on the soles) and legs.

- 'Glove or stocking' distribution of injuries on hands or feet and ankles with no splash marks and a clear edge where there has been forced immersion.

- Regular edges to injured area.

- Depth of injuries – may be full thickness.

- 'Hole in the doughnut' scald – centre of the buttocks is spared when child is forcibly immersed in scalding water.

- Splash scalds may be seen in accidental scalds. However they may also be seen when hot liquid has been thrown deliberately.

- Cigarette burns — accidentally inflicted burns are usually associated with a circular mark and a tail. Deliberately inflicted burns are usually deep and tend to scar.

- Differential diagnoses — skin disease or infection, e.g. impetigo, severe nappy rash; unusual circumstances, e.g. hot metal seatbelt buckles; immobility or altered pain perception because of neurological conditions such as cerebral palsy or congenital insensitivity to pain.

Bites

- Animal bites result in puncturing, cutting and tearing of the skin.

- Human bites result in bruising, usually crescent-shaped. Individual tooth marks may be seen. Breaking of the skin is not usual unless the bite has been very forceful. However, the appearances of bite marks can be distorted by the contours of the area bitten and by movement when the bite occurs.

- Distinguishing between a child and adult bite can be difficult and the assistance of a forensic odontologist or dentist may be helpful.

Fractures

- May be the presenting feature of child abuse but may also be discovered during assessment of other clinical signs and symptoms.

- Non-accidental fractures may not be detected except by radiology, e.g. rib fractures in a young child.

- May present to GP as reluctance to move or non-movement of a limb, or limping, or with swelling and pain with no or little explanation.

- Assessment for possible fractures and association with child abuse is best done by radiologists together with paediatricians. Relevant information about the child and family that the GP and primary healthcare team have should be shared with these colleagues and with social services.

Poisoning/suffocation/submersion

- Children may ingest harmful substances because of lack of supervision, deliberate self-harm or inappropriate administration by a carer.

- Non-accidental poisoning can be difficult to identify but can have serious consequences. Presenting features are usually in the category of 'fits, faints and funny turns', are unexplained, and may be recurrent.

- Non-accidental suffocation may present like cot death but presentations may also be in the category of 'fits, faints and funny turns' that are unexplained.

- Non-accidental submersion may not be easy to identify. The victims are usually toddlers and the history may be inconsistent and changing. There is often a history of maternal mental illness or of the child being left with an inappropriate carer. There may be other signs of abuse.

- Such children are usually referred to paediatricians but GPs have a role in contributing to the assessment because of their knowledge of the family, e.g. if there are parental mental health problems, prescriptions of potential poisons for members of the household, previous unexplained deaths.

Factitious illness/Munchausen Syndrome by Proxy

- In this form of abuse a child is presented with an illness that is fabricated by the parent/carer. There are repeated presentations for medical assessments, investigations and treatment. The perpetrator usually denies any knowledge of the aetiology of the illness. The child's symptoms and signs disappear when she/he is separated from the perpetrator.

- The symptoms and signs may be invented or the child may be directly subjected to harm by the perpetrator attempting to produce these, e.g. causing apnoea attacks by suffocation (*see* section above on poisoning/suffocation/submersion) or the child given medication such as insulin to produce altered consciousness. Investigation results may be tampered with, e.g. blood may be added to urine, stools or vomit, or temperature recordings may be manipulated to suggest fever.

- The GP may be the first person to become concerned that a child is being harmed in this way, although it is more usual that the child is referred for paediatric assessment of her/his symptoms and signs. It may be some time before the possibility of factitious illness is considered.

- However, GPs have a role in contributing to strategy discussions and assessments of the child and family in these situations because of their knowledge of the family and the information held in their records.

Sexual abuse

The following situations are strongly associated with child sexual abuse.

- Statement from child – this should always be taken seriously and recorded verbatim if possible. It is important that the child is not questioned in too much detail but only sufficiently to establish that sexual abuse is the issue (*see* Chapter 12).

- Sexually transmitted diseases — when this is diagnosed in a child, sexual abuse must be considered.
- Pregnancy.
- Sexualised behaviour or inappropriate sexual knowledge.
- Bruising and/or signs of injury in the genital area, inner aspect of thighs, lower abdomen or pubic area. 'Love bites' are of concern.

The following situations are less specific but sexual abuse should be considered in the differential diagnosis:

- Symptoms of local trauma or infection, e.g. vaginal discharge, perineal soreness, genital and/or rectal bleeding, anal trauma or genital warts.
- Symptoms related to emotional effects, e.g. enuresis, encopresis, loss of concentration, loss of appetite, sleeping difficulties, self-harm, change in behaviour and/or school performance, recurrent abdominal pains/headaches.

Often there are no abnormal physical findings.

Neglect

This category of abuse is harm brought about by omission rather than commission. There are overlaps between this category and that of emotional abuse.

- Inappropriate or inadequate parenting, for example:
  - affecting the physical state of the child, such as failure to thrive, inadequate hygiene, appearance of 'deprivation

hands and feet'. Deprivation hands and feet were described by Glover *et al.* in 1985. Deep pink (sometimes with a bluish tinge), mildly oedematous hands and feet were seen in a group of children living in families with considerable deprivation. Such an appearance may give rise to concern about the child's cardiac status
 — repeated attendance for minor injuries, especially to different sources of medical advice such as GPs, A&E departments, the health visitor, the practice nurse
 — repeated failure to keep or make medical appointments.

- Refusal to seek or to co-operate with appropriate medical advice — in some situations it is obvious that a child will be harmed, e.g. if medical treatment such as insulin for diabetes, or TB treatment, is refused. Other instances that are not so extreme, e.g. repeated failures to attend for treatment of hearing difficulty, could be neglectful and consideration must be given as to whether the child's health and development to his/her full potential is being harmed.

Emotional abuse

The following dimensions of emotionally abusive relationships have been described by Glaser (1993: 251–67).

- Persistent negative attitudes of the parent to the child, leading to rejection and harsh punishment/discipline, e.g. persistent blaming of the child, belittling the child, terrorising the child with threats of severe physical punishment or threats of abandonment, isolating the child in confined or frightening situations.

- Promoting insecure attachment by conditional parenting, e.g. the parent will continue to care only if the child continues to be good/grateful.

- Emotional unavailability or neglect of the child.

- Inappropriate developmental expectations, e.g. failure to protect or overprotecting, parents expecting child to fit in with the adults' needs, blaming the child.

- Failure to recognise child's individuality and psychological boundaries.

- Cognitive distortions and inconsistencies, e.g. inconsistent parental expectations, unpredictable parental responses.

- The child/young person may present with symptoms such as enuresis, encopresis, loss of concentration/short attention span, loss of appetite, sleeping difficulties, self-harm, change in behaviour and/or school performance, difficult behaviour, low self-esteem.

The GP and members of the primary healthcare team may be well placed to observe and have knowledge of family relationships and dynamics which could alert them to the possibility that a child is being emotionally abused and/or neglected.

Key features of emotional abuse and neglect (from Skuse 1997) are as follows.

In infants:

- physical
  - failure to thrive
  - recurrent and persistent minor infections
  - repeated attendances at A&E departments and/or hospital admissions
  - unexplained bruising
  - severe nappy rash

- developmental
  - general delay

- behavioural
  - attachment disorders (*see* Chapter 13): anxiety, avoidance, social unresponsiveness.

In preschool children:

- physical
  - short, may be underweight
  - microcephaly
  - unkempt and dirty

- developmental
  - language delayed
  - short attention span
  - social and emotional immaturity

- behavioural
  - overactive
  - aggressive and impulsive
  - indiscriminate friendliness
  - seeks physical contact from strangers.

In school children:

- physical
  - short stature, may be underweight
  - poor hygiene
  - unkempt appearance

- developmental
  - learning difficulties
  - low self-esteem
  - short attention span
  - poor coping skills
  - social and emotional immaturity

- behavioural
  - poor relationships
  - aggressive, overactive, destructive
  - lacks confidence, withdrawn
  - poor school performance
  - wetting, soiling.

In teenagers:

- physical
  - short, may be under- or overweight
  - poor general health
  - delayed puberty
  - unkempt appearance
  - poor hygiene

- developmental
  - school failure

- behavioural
  - school non-attendance
  - destructive (to self, others, property)
  - risk-taking behaviours – smoking, alcohol, drugs, sexual promiscuity
  - lying, stealing
  - runaway.

References

Department of Health (1999) *Working Together to Safeguard Children.* The Stationery Office, London.

Glaser D (1993) Emotional abuse. In: Hobbs CJ and Wynne JM (eds) *Balliere's Clinical Paediatrics International Practice* vol. 1, no. 1, ch. 13. Balliere Tindall, London.

Glover S, Nicoll A and Pullan C (1985) Deprivation hands and feet. *Arch Dis Child.* **60**: 976–7.

Skuse D (1997) Emotional abuse and neglect. In: Meadow R (ed) *ABC of Child Abuse* (3e). BMJ Publishing Group, London.

Further reading

Hobbs CJ, Hanks HGI and Wynne JM (1999) *Child Abuse and Neglect. A Clinician's Handbook* (2e). Churchill Livingstone, London.

12
Action to take following recognition

Yin Ng

What to do when child abuse is diagnosed/suspected

First of all, do not panic. Remember that your local Area Child Protection Committee will have procedures based on *Working Together to Safeguard Children* (DoH 1999), of which you will have knowledge and which you will be expected to follow. The nurse members of the primary healthcare team will be given similar guidance.

Secondly, you should be able to discuss difficult or worrying cases with your local senior paediatrician/designated doctor in child protection (*see* Chapter 3), senior GP colleagues or social services.

There is an expectation that if you are told of abuse or if you strongly suspect it, then you will have to make a child protection referral to social services. It is good practice to inform the parents/carer/child that you are doing so (*see* Chapter 5 for additional considerations in sexual abuse). This can be a difficult area for GPs, who are reluctant to damage their relationship with other family members.

Thirdly, making an enquiry of the local child protection register (*see* Chapter 9) is essential as it is another way of sharing information and concerns about a particular child or family. The lack of information should not deter you from making a referral to social services if you consider that the child has been or is being abused.

Effective communication is essential. Verbal discussions and referrals must be confirmed in writing to minimise confusion and misunderstandings.

Physical abuse

Serious injury

A child requiring hospital treatment and/or investigations such as X-rays will need to be admitted to hospital with the relevant information shared with hospital colleagues. The GP needs to make a child protection referral to the appropriate social services team as soon as possible. The referral should be confirmed in writing with a copy taken for the medical notes.

Injuries not requiring treatment

If abuse is strongly suspected then the GP must make a referral to social services. If abuse is suspected but you would like advice, there will be a local arrangement whereby you can discuss matters such as where the child could be seen for a second opinion if this seems the best course of action. In all cases it must be remembered that it is the welfare and safety of the child (and other children in the household) which is paramount.

Sexual abuse

A clear statement to you of sexual abuse must be referred to social services and/or to the police, according to local child protection procedures. Similarly, allegations of sexual abuse should also be referred, as health professionals do not have the statutory duties of investigation.

Remember not to ask too detailed questions as the child will be interviewed later by the investigating professionals and there is a danger of affecting the evidence. Ask only what is necessary to determine the nature of the abuse and to find out if the child needs urgent medical treatment.

However, as discussed in Chapter 5, it is not always appropriate to be open with the child's carer/parent about this kind of referral, as there may be collusion between the carer/parent and the perpetrator. Knowledge that a referral is being made may put the child at risk of further harm from pressure to retract her/his allegation/statement. It must be emphasised that it is important to acknowledge to the child that you have heard what she/he has told you and that you will act on it. This can be a difficult area when the young person tells you that she/he does not wish you to tell anyone else.

If you are concerned that sexual abuse may be happening because of symptoms and/or signs or your knowledge of the social circumstances, it is necessary to discuss this with other members of the primary healthcare team, the local school nurse and community paediatrician, depending on circumstances. It may also be helpful to discuss your concerns with your local senior paediatrician/designated doctor in child protection or senior GP colleagues, or with social services to decide whether a referral under the child protection procedures is appropriate at this stage.

Medical examination by a GP in cases of sexual abuse should usually be limited to:

- assessing and managing any acute injuries or medical problem appropriately within the role of the GP

- excluding gross pathology if the parents/child request an examination.

It is now usual practice that children and young people who have suffered or are alleged to have suffered sexual abuse are examined jointly by police surgeons/forensic examiners and paediatricians who undertake such examinations regularly (often these are community paediatricians). The aim is for children to be examined once only where possible. The local child protection procedures will give guidance on this.

Neglect and emotional abuse

Concerns about neglect and/or emotional abuse should be discussed and information shared with other members of the primary healthcare team and with other involved health professionals. There should be a local arrangement for you to discuss your concerns also with a senior paediatrician/GP/designated doctor and also with social services. The preparation of a chronology of events/incidents, although a time-consuming task, can be extremely useful in assessing whether there is significant harm.

Case examples

Case 1

A five-year-old attends for his pre-school booster immunisation. The practice nurse notices bruises on his upper arm and is suspicious of how they were caused. In accordance with your practice guidelines, she asks for your advice.

Response to Case 1

- Ask for an explanation.
- Examine the whole child.

- If the explanation given doesn't fit the findings:
  - Explain that you have concerns that the explanation does not fit the injuries observed.
  - Explain that under these circumstances it is necessary to get further advice and another opinion and that you have no choice but to make a referral to social services in order for this to be carried out.
  - Check the child protection register.
  - Document clearly in the case notes and follow up your telephone referral by letter, keeping a copy in the notes.
  - It would also be helpful to discuss this child with your health visitor.

Case 2

A three-year-old girl is brought to the GP by her father because of some blistering on her trunk. There is an area of redness with the appearance of a scald or burn on her abdomen.

Response to Case 2

- On examination, the appearance is consistent with a burn or a scald.

- Previous discussion with the health visitor had identified some concerns about neglect.

- Explain that you have concerns and need to refer to social services (follow up in writing).

- Social services ask for the child to be seen by a paediatrician. By this time, satellite lesions have appeared and a diagnosis of impetigo is made.

- Because of concerns about the general level of care for the child, extra input from the health visitor is arranged, and the family receive help in the care of the child.

Case 3

A family consisting of a mother and six young children have recently moved into the area and register with the practice. The mother complains of feeling depressed and presents one of the children with difficult behaviour. The mother's partner, who is also registered with the practice, asks for help with his drug habit and aggressive outbursts. What do you do?

Response to Case 3

- Discuss with the health visitor and ensure that the notes are obtained from their previous practice as quickly as possible — both medical and health visiting notes. If possible, contact the previous GP.

- In view of the link between domestic violence, drug abuse and child protection issues, it would be a good idea to check the child protection register of the area that the child previously lived in.

- Explore reasons as to why the mother is depressed and take a full history about the child with difficult behaviour.

- Enlist health visitor involvement.

- Also take a full history from the partner and make a mental link between drug abuse, domestic violence and child protection issues.

- Refer him for help with drug addiction and aggression. In order to help with the assessment, the team/doctor receiving the referral needs to be aware that the patient is living with a partner and six children.

- Consider making a note of family links of the mother's depression and the father's aggression and drug problem on all paediatric family members' notes.

- Meet regularly with the health visitor and consider referral to social services as a 'child in need' (*see* Chapter 2), depending on circumstances.

- If there are children of school age in the family, liaise with the local school health team to share relevant information.

This type of case needs constant monitoring and good communication by the whole team.

Case 4

A two-year-old girl shows very slow growth and some developmental delay. She should be attending the ENT outpatients department (previous grommets) and eye clinic (squint) for follow-up but there is a history of recurrent non-attendances there and also at the surgery. What do you do?

Response to Case 4

- Share your concerns with the parent/carer.

- Discuss with the health visitor.

- Discuss with/refer to local (community) paediatrician for assessment of growth and development, including your concerns about non-attendances and any relevant knowledge of the family.

- If in addition there are concerns about level of care or knowledge about previous child protection concerns, discuss with social services and make a referral — possibly under Section 17 'child in need' (*see* Chapter 2) if considered appropriate.

A case like this requires continuing review and co-ordination, which the GP may be best placed to do.

Case 5

A 13-year-old girl comes to see you complaining of abdominal pain. She is accompanied by her mother but, when offered the choice, she indicates that she wants to be seen by herself. She tells you that she is being sexually abused by her stepfather. What do you do?

Response to Case 5

Following this disclosure of the abuse to you, it is important to acknowledge that you have heard and understood what has been said. Indicate that the best way to get help is to enlist the assistance of social services, and explain that someone will visit. It is not appropriate to take a detailed history or do an examination, nor is it appropriate to tell the mother what has been said unless the child explicitly asks you to do this. Make sure that your referral is followed up in writing.

Case 6

A mother brings her five-year-old daughter to your surgery. She is concerned that the babysitter (a male aged 16) did something of a sexual nature to her child. The mother asks you to examine her daughter 'to make sure she is alright'.

Response to Case 6

It is important to reassure the mother that she has taken the right action by coming to see you. Then you can explain that the way forward is for you to refer the problem to social services who will look into the matter. You should explain that a police surgeon and possibly a paediatrician together (depending on local procedures) will then examine the child, so that the child is examined only once. However, if there is concern of injury, or the mother still would like her child examined by you, provided the child consents it is appropriate to inspect the genitalia. Follow up the referral in writing and document all details in the notes.

Case 7

A mother and grandmother bring a six-month-old baby to your surgery because they want him to be checked over following an episode when the father grabbed him from the mother and shook him to stop him crying. You are aware that there is a volatile and aggressive relationship between his parents. The baby looks well. What do you do?

Response to Case 7

Clearly the baby needs to be examined, but even if the examination is normal the child needs referral to hospital for a brain scan and skeletal survey and also needs referring to social services. Mother and grandmother need to be aware that you are making a referral. Explain that you understand the problems of stress within the family under the circumstances. Document your action in the notes, and follow up the referral in writing.

The injuries that infants may suffer from being shaken are well-documented, e.g. fractured ribs, subdural haemorrhage and effusions, and cerebral injuries. However, there is still little awareness of the dangers of shaking babies. In a number of districts around the country there have been various awareness-raising campaigns, e.g. the 'Don't Shake the Baby' campaign in

Nottinghamshire, supported by the ACPC. There are also information pages in the parent-held child health record. Protocols for assessing possible shaking injuries are in place in some areas.

References

Department of Health (1999) *Working Together to Safeguard Children.* The Stationery Office, London.

13
Implications of abuse for the child

Rachel Leheup

The model of physical injury has been unhelpful for considering longer-term effects and psychological consequences of abuse. It has encouraged us to think of child abuse as a series of incidents needing short-term investigation rather than a process that may require longer intervention.

Childhood is the time that the brain is developing at the fastest rate in all areas and the cumulative effects of living with neglect, violence and physical and sexual abuse can have an effect on one or more aspects of the child's functioning. Recent advances in technology have allowed the study of the growth in neuro-synaptic pathways in infants and young children and it has been shown that being reared in chaos, neglect and violence results in disorganised and underdeveloped brains (Perry *et al.* 1995). In young children, this tends to lead to either hyper-arousal with a fight/flight response, or dissociation where the child seems unresponsive, numb or cut off.

Adults often misunderstand these reactions and the child is seen as disordered or defiant. The responses evoked by the child's behaviour reinforce the fear and consolidate the coping mechanisms, so setting up the vicious cycle that is commonly present in chronic abuse. As time goes on, if the situation does not improve, a range of difficulties can emerge. These symptoms can be seen to arise out of coping strategies the child has employed to live with and accommodate to the abuse.

There are no specific symptoms associated with child abuse and different types of abuse do not produce different syndromes. The fear, loss of trust and distortions of their closest relationships are present in all forms of abuse and are the components that influence long-term development.

The prevalence of a degree of the various forms of abuse is high, but the overall figures are impossible to ascertain as much goes undiscovered (*see* Chapter 4).

Any study of socially marginalised young people, for example, runaways, those who self-harm, substance misusers, persistent offenders and those with mental health problems, have a very high rate of reported abuse. However, it is important to remember that a number of children who are abused do not go on to display major difficulties.

The difficulties shown by a child depend on their age and developmental level when the abuse began, and their innate temperament and resilience. The presence of other factors in the environment interacts with these difficulties to mitigate or accentuate the problems. Anna Freud (1976) points out that there is no one-to-one relationship between adverse parenting and the distortions that might arise in the child's development – cruel treatment can produce either an aggressive and violent, or a timid, crushed and passive being.

The developmental outcome is determined not by an environmental interference *per se*, but by its interaction with the inborn and acquired resources of the child.

Recent work has moved away from a dichotomy between either genetic and neuro-physiological reasons or psychosocial ones as the cause of behaviour problems. Pre- and post-natal influences of both types affect the brain and this has an effect on the behaviour of the child, which in turn affects the response from others.

Cognitive effects

Learning can be impaired as the direct result of an under-stimulating or abusive environment. The ability to learn can also be impaired by the effort necessary not to think or talk about the abuse that is occurring (Bowlby 1979).

The language of maltreated children tends to develop slower than in their non-abused counterparts, and abused children also have fewer ways of describing feelings. Impaired language development prevents the acquisition of the symbolic and abstract thought necessary to learn in school.

Overactivity, poor concentration and troublesome behaviour compound cognitive difficulties by making school placement and academic achievement difficult.

Psychological effects

It is important to remember that most child abuse happens within the family. This is a betrayal of the core relationships a child needs to develop, and very basic psychological functions like trust, attachment and a sense of self-identity are compromised.

John Bowlby studied the relationships between infants and their primary caregivers, usually their mothers (Bowlby 1989). This first relationship with an attachment figure becomes the blueprint from which the child develops other relationships. As work on attachment behaviours has been expanded, there is a greater understanding of how difficulties in early attachment can lead to problem behaviours later. The minute day-to-day interplay between an infant and carer gives rise to trust and an ability to control inner feelings if things are going well. Secure attachment allows a young child to develop self-esteem and empathy.

When studied closely, other forms of attachment can be described (Ainsworth 1985).

- Inconsistent caring gives rise to **ambivalent** attachment where the child wants their carer but resists the comfort offered.

- Unresponsiveness in the carer, commonly due to depression or substance misuse, leads to **avoidance** attachment where the child does not look to the parent for reassurance and shows little emotional response to the parent's coming and going. This avoidance pattern can later lead to depression, substance misuse, self-harming and bulimia.

- Abusive parenting, where the main caregiver is also the source of harm, gives rise to **disorganised** attachment where the child approaches the parent in a distorted, disorganised way. The child might freeze or stare into space. Children with this type of attachment pattern are particularly vulnerable to further problems within and outside the family. Their relationship with their peers is difficult and it is hard for them to make close, trusting relationships. This has serious implications if they are placed outside the family, as it may be hard for them to gain positive experiences from an alternative placement.

Other behavioural effects

Many abused children have low self-esteem and this can interfere with their taking advantage of good experiences that could help to mitigate the effects of abuse. They do not think they deserve to be well treated or respected. The inability to contain strong emotions internally, and the way these early relationships affect brain development, can lead to impulsive, poorly controlled behaviour, which is often aggressive. It is not uncommon to meet young people in the criminal justice system that have an early history of severe abuse.

All of these behavioural problems lead to unrewarding contact with adults and peers and validate the child's view, developed through abuse, that she or he is unlovable and bad and the world is a dangerous place.

Intervention

Although the effect of abuse on children's neuro-psychological development can be profound, it is important not to take a position of despair. The brain is a plastic organ and patterns of thinking and behaviour can change. Violence towards children is a culturally embedded phenomenon, not a disease, so the interventions need to be social as well as professional. Society has periods of recognising child maltreatment and then forgetting again. Our current interest only began with Kempe's work 40 years ago (Kempe *et al.* 1962).

The best intervention is prevention. All professionals involved with children should promote child-centred policies, including those addressing family poverty, racism, poor housing, and poor schools. Social forces that allow the victimisation of those with less social power result in high rates of child maltreatment (Briere 1992).

Secondary prevention involves targeting vulnerable groups so that the number of positive and neutral experiences the child has is increased. Current DoH recommendations in child protection work recommend moving from only dealing with major events of abuse towards a broader-based service for 'children in need'. Ideally this would offer family and child support when families are under pressure and are seen to be vulnerable, rather than waiting until problems have occurred. Government initiatives under the social exclusion policies, such as Sure Start, should go some way towards meeting these ideas. Sure Start provides families living in areas of social exclusion with a child under four years with a trained volunteer to help them develop positive parenting of their children. The ability to regain some pleasure, fun and play with children is a good way to help them develop their potential. A similar programme in America in the 1960s, called Headstart, was shown to make a significant difference to the children at long-term follow-up, especially with regard to educational attainment and employment.

Effects of abuse in childhood on adult development

Untreated trauma arising from abuse contributes heavily to mental health and social problems, not just in childhood but into adult life. Adults can have great difficulty creating and sustaining intimate, personal relationships, which can lead to sexual and marital difficulties (McCann and Pearlman 1990). This can then go on to make parenting difficulties for the next generation. For some, the early effects on their brain and emotional development means they are impulsive, aggressive, have learning difficulties, get excluded from school and go on to become delinquents and substance misusers. This pattern of behaviour has been repeatedly shown to be very persistent if there are no mitigating factors and the children go on to be parents who rear their children in similar ways.

The children who are more withdrawn and internalise the emotional distress are likely to go on to develop mental health problems. Patterns of deliberate self-harm, eating disorders, depression, anxiety and personality disorders consume large amounts of resources and professional time, often to little avail as the link between their symptoms and their childhood experiences of abuse are not made and the interventions offered not helpful. Post-Traumatic Stress Disorder is now thought to be a significant consequence in some cases of abuse and may give rise to symptoms that can be mistaken for a developing psychosis.

The recent debate initiated by the Government about the smacking of children and the meaning of 'reasonable chastisement' has again confirmed our cultural acceptance of the aggression and exploitation embedded in the way we rear our children. It hampers our ability to recognise parent–child difficulties early on and to manage them in a sensitive way. The connection between child maltreatment and later dysfunctional behaviours therefore gets overlooked in spite of the body of evidence supporting the connection.

We need to develop a broad framework within which to address the spectrum of child abuse and its consequences. Professional groups and agencies can overcome their differences and contribute together towards effective intervention in this difficult field.

References

Ainsworth MDS (1985) Patterns of infant–mother attachment and effect on development. *Bulletin of the New York Academy of Sciences.* **61**: 771–91.

Bowlby J (1979) On knowing what you're not supposed to know and feeling what you're not supposed to feel. *Canadian Journal of Psychiatry.* **24/5**: 403–8.

Bowlby J (1989) *A Secure Basis.* Tavistock/Routledge, London.

Briere J (1992) *Child Abuse Trauma.* Sage, London.

Freud A (1976) Psychopathology seen against the background of normal development. *British Journal of Psychiatry.* **129**: 401–6.

Kempe CH, Silverman FN, Steele BF, Droegmuller W and Silver HK (1962) The battered child syndrome. *JAMA.* **181**: 17–24.

McCann IL and Pearlman LA (1990) *Psychological Trauma and the Adult Survivor: Theory, Therapy and Transformation.* Brunner/Mazel, New York.

Perry BD, Pollard RA, Blakley TL and Vigilante D (1995) Childhood trauma, the neurobiology of adaptation, and 'use-dependent' development of the brain: how 'states become traits'. *Infant Mental Health Journal* **16**(4): 271–90.

Index